The Fall In Love Process: Body Program

Stop Treating Your Body Like It's A Bad Boyfriend

Dr. Lauren Sierra Thomas

Order this book online at www.trafford.com
or email orders@trafford.com

Most Trafford titles are also available at major online book retailers.

Printed in the United States of America.

ISBN: 978-1-4251-7453-8 (sc)
ISBN: 978-1-4669-5111-2 (hc)
ISBN: 978-1-4669-5110-5 (e)

Trafford rev. 11/09/2012

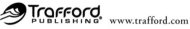

www.trafford.com

North America & international
toll-free: 1 888 232 4444 (USA & Canada)
phone: 250 383 6864 • fax: 812 355 4082

CONTENTS

You Wouldn't Exist Without Your Body
The Fall In Love (FIL) Body Program & How It Began
A Message For You
A Note To Men

Chapter One
**Women & Their Bodies:
A Silent Epidemic Of Suffering**...................................... 1

The Current Body Paradigm That Keeps You Insecure & Anxious
The Beauty Industry—The Billion Dollar Machine
     That Plays You Like A Puppet On A String
Not A Campaign Against Beauty
Why Do I Need To Change?
What Makes The Fall In Love Body Program Unique?
The Key To Why Diets & Exercise Fail
Women's Relationship With Food
The Real Reason You Want A "Perfect" Body
Self-Betrayal & Empowered Choice

Witnessing: A Process For Self Awareness
How To Make Affirmations More Effective
The Power of Appreciation
What Promotes Healing?

Chapter Five
Mind-Body Healing Techniques:
Access & Change Your Unconscious Beliefs

Emotional Freedom Technique (EFT) In A Nutshell
PSYCH-K: Access & Change Your Unconscious Beliefs

Conclusions

You Are God To Your Cells
The Answers Lie Within:
    The Gods on Mount Olympus Hide The Secret of Life

Appendix A
The Exercises

Core Exercise One:
    Everything I Experienced Today
Core Exercise Two:
    My Body And All It Does For Me
Core Exercise Three:
    My Favorite Moments In Life
Anchoring

DEDICATION

This book is dedicated to Ruth Lee of Madera, a wise and remarkable woman who passed me the toilet paper in a public restroom. As a result of our fateful encounter, and at her prompting, I embarked on the path of writing.

The memory of Ruth shall be etched in my heart and soul forever.

IMPORTANT NOTE TO THE READER

The ideas and suggestions in this book are not meant to be used in place of sound medical or therapeutic advice and treatment. If you have conditions that merit the use of a medical and/or mental health practitioner or therapist, it is essential that you seek such aid.

ACKNOWLEDGMENTS

My first acknowledgment goes to my former boyfriend who told me he was no longer attracted to me because of my weight gain. He gave me the gift of an awakening in my heart and soul that enabled me to embrace and fall in love with my body!

Lenny Prosseda, my lifelong friend and business advisor, the person who's assisted me through everything with his knowledge, humor, and wisdom—and the one who has always believed in me. I could not have done it without you. You mean the world to me.

I wish to thank my remarkable friend Dr. Heather Greenwald for her generous words. My life is enriched by our friendship.

Greg Dewitt, webmaster for my BestRelationshipsEver site, my heartfelt thank you. You did so much for so little out of generosity and because you believed in my vision. You are a wonderful human being.

Many thanks to Yvonne Brett for her fine editing. My book was improved greatly as a result.

To my dear, precious friends. You know who you are. I am constantly sustained and held in love by you, you amazing critters. Your love nourishes me and I find passion for life because of it. Tons of kisses and hugs to you.

Last, but not least, my family. You mean everything to me. My heart is filled with love for you and is with you always. I shall love you throughout eternity!

FOREWORD

There are people who change our lives. They listen to you and hear what you are saying and understand you. They get it. They get you. They care about you. When you find one of these people, listen to them. They tell you what you need to hear, sometimes far afield of what you wanted to hear, yet always with compassion. Dr. Thomas does this. She has gained perspective from training and experience as a respected and gifted psychologist and as a great woman and true friend.

Although Dr. Thomas holds a doctorate and two master's degrees, her real treasure is in the wisdom acquired through a life fully lived. She has an uncanny ability to develop models to help others that are a result of her own life experiences. She has learned along the way and we get to benefit.

In her career as a psychologist she has worked with some of the most violent criminals in our country and she has identified in this book a far greater danger among us. Dr. Thomas sees the torrential storm women trudge through and offers a way to a clear vantage. In that clarity there is a new air and new breath.

Lauren's words change you, because they are real, they are outside the regular, beyond the flow of familiar and they thoughtfully remind you what your insides know that you politely ignore. She is insightful and it is delivered with an irreverence that tells you not to be quite so serious. She is the kind of person that can tell you to do it differently and you do. She has changed the lives of her patients, her clients, her students, her family and her friends. I am honored to include myself in her circle of friends and can tell you she once gave me a piece of sage advice for which I will always be grateful. You have just become part of a great person's circle of influence. I am so excited for you. If you ever get the chance to meet her, do, she is as great as she seems.

Dr. Heather Greenwald
Chief Psychologist
CDCR

the Fall in Love Process
www.thefallinloveprocess.com
xvi

PREFACE

The Fall In Love Process (FIL)

The *FIL Process* is a roadmap for you to have everything your heart truly desires. Everything you want in your life—whether it be a great body, a relationship, family, job, or house—is because you believe in the having of it you will feel good. *The Fall In Love Process* helps you learn how to feel good. Isn't that the real "prize"?

Unlike what you are promised by many "experts", I am not going to pretend that *The FIL Process* will magically eliminate every bad hair moment or day of your life. Not only is that kind of transcendence perspective a myth, but holding that as something you can attain sets you up for failure and a sense of disappointment in yourself.

We are not robots. We need a little wiggle room to be human. Yet, we also need tools to help us feel good about our lives. We need new ways of looking at life that ease our pain and disappointment, assist us in viewing things differently, and help us to feel better. We need the comfort of a sense that someone is in our corner and that we have a soft place to land.

Think about *The Fall In Love Process* like this: if you can feel significantly better about your body, yourself, your love relationships, and your break-ups, isn't that a ride worth taking?

The Fall In Love Process is about falling in love with your life and includes three core programs that will help you manage and feel good in the following areas:

Loving Your Body (Body Program)
Loving Your Self/Love Relationships (Relationship Program)
Loving Separation (Break-Up Program)

The Fall In Love Body Program helps you to fall in love with your body. Welcome to *The Body Program* and *The Fall In Love Process.*

HOW TO USE THIS BOOK

You may use this book in a variety of ways. One way, of course, is to read straight through the book in its entirety. I recommend this approach, as it will enable you to gain a complete overview and help you understand the concepts that you are applying.

It is not a necessity, however, to use FIL in this manner. You may find that you do not have a particular interest in the introduction or how the program came into being, for example.

I would recommend that you *begin the core written exercises in the Appendix immediately*, as you do not need to understand all the concepts in the book for the exercises to be helpful.

If you would like, you may proceed to the exercises and begin—and even conclude—there. The exercises in themselves are enough to promote change in your life. In fact, **the exercises are the core of FIL as they reframe how you feel about your body.** Applying these few exercises can facilitate profound transformation in your life and in your relationship with your body. The core exercises are simple and yet profound. Do not underestimate them and do not skip them.

You might decide to read the entire book first and then begin the exercises. The important thing is to begin.

I do recommend that you read the entire program, since it lays a foundation for the concepts underlying the exercises. Understanding how the concepts developed provides an integral understanding of the exercises, and should help to anchor your understanding, as well as provide inspiration. The point is to create an emotion, which is very important in making a change in your life. A thought without emotion is not particularly effective.

FIL teaches you how to shift your whole perspective of how you think and feel about your body. You will learn to question your current beliefs and choose more empowering ones, and will be given several tools and techniques for personal growth and transformation.

You may be introduced to some ideas or assumptions that are new to you. If so, choose to keep an open and receptive mind. You may not relate to, understand, or agree with all the concepts introduced or the assumptions stated. That is actually good. This program will still work for you. It is not necessary to relate to, or even agree with, every aspect of *FIL*. Questioning and developing your own beliefs makes you your own individual. I would ask though, that you attempt to remain open-minded as you are reading the book and exploring the exercises.

It may happen that you read some parts of the program—especially those relating to how amazing your body is, the uniqueness of you as a human being, and the wonderment of life itself—and initially have a negative reaction. If you are not feeling good about your body, yourself, or your life, at first it can almost seem like reading these things is like rubbing salt into an open wound. It can feel painful because you are not in a good feeling place.

If you have a negative reaction, recognize that this is why you are reading and using *Fall In Love*—to develop inspiration about your body, your uniqueness, and to begin to feel better about your life.

Falling In Love is a process. Be gentle with yourself. Stay with it and watch what arises. We will be working with your thoughts and feelings about your body. Be open. Change can and does happen.

If you have been engaged in personal growth work for some time and a few of the concepts are familiar, that's great. It always helps to reinforce what we already know on some level.

Sometimes it takes hearing something several times, or perhaps having it expressed in a slightly different way, to have it really sink in and become a useful tool that we can incorporate into our lives. Certain concepts which are critical will be repeated for this reason.

In either case—whether you have never heard of the concepts or are very familiar with some of them—I hope that you remain open and willing to expand into a new way of viewing your body and your life. *Fall In Love* is **unique** in its approach to healing your relationship with your body.

I am happy to share this information with you, in the strong belief that it may benefit you, enrich your life, and increase your well-being and happiness exponentially.

ABOUT THE EXERCISES

Do **not** skip the exercises.

The exercises are central to the *Fall In Love Body Program* and form the foundation for loving your body. It is where you begin to actually practice new ways of thinking about and viewing your body.

Doing the exercises is what will help you most to become a person who loves and appreciates your body. The purpose of the written exercises is to replace negative messages and feelings about your body with more positive and life-affirming ones.

The exercises are aimed at not only getting you to *think* about loving your body, but also to *feel* it deeply in the core of your being. Affirmations are not effective if you're just reciting words. You need to *feel* them and *imagine how you will feel when they actualize in order for them to be effective.*

The exercises are aimed at helping you begin to recognize and get in touch with the tremendous service your body provides for you as it carries you through this life.

In fact, the purpose of these exercises is to help you realize that you would not be here, nor would you have *any* life experiences without your body. **You as you know you would not exist without your body.** I don't know about you, but I find this remarkable.

The exercises form the foundation of the active role you will take in healing yourself and befriending your body. ***If you can only do one thing, do the exercises.*** These exercises are the way you reframe what you believe and how you feel about your body.

I truly believe that if you complete these exercises daily, as instructed, you will experience a significant shift in perspective toward your body. You will never again experience your body in quite the same way. I believe you will feel tremendously more appreciative toward your body and it will respond to your appreciation.

the Fall in Love Process
www.thefallinloveprocess.com
xxiv

INTRODUCTION

*What is this body? That shadow of a shadow that somehow
contains the entire universe.*

—Rumi

Think about the reason why you want the things you want. *What is behind your wanting?* The real reason you want anything is because you believe that in the having of that thing you will feel better and be happier.

What is behind your yearning as a woman to have a good body? You believe you will be valued and loved more as a human being if you have an attractive body. You may not have ever thought of it in this way, but most likely that is what is at the core of your wanting a great body.

The anxiety, shame, and pain you currently feel over your body is connected to your feeling less valuable or lovable when it doesn't meet the societal standard.

Ironically, even if your body does meet that standard you may still feel anxious, self-conscious, and worried; fearful that your body isn't good enough or that it may betray you at any moment. At best, your body ages.

The FIL Body Program is here to provide a roadmap for you to change at a core level how you perceive, what you believe, and how you feel about your body. But that's not all.

Most importantly, it is to address *the real reason you want anything*: to feel better. Since this is why you want anything, it is important that you learn tools and techniques to get to that end result: feeling good in your life.

Feeling better does not have to be tied to a specific outcome. *Notice, the ultimate desire is to feel good. Learning how to create that feeling in your life is what you really want.* And that's the journey we'll be taking together.

The Body Program is specifically focused on helping you feel better about your body, while learning some tools to help you feel good in other areas of your life as well.

You Wouldn't Exist Without Your Body

As obvious as it is that you would not exist in this life without your body, have you ever really considered it? Have you ever even noticed what your body does for you daily? Have you ever offered your body appreciation for all it does to keep you functioning so that you can have a life?

How is it that as a culture we have given almost no attention to this critical piece of basic information? We have not been trained to notice. Instead we have been taught to criticize this magnificent operating system that enables us to be alive.

In fact, the barrage of criticism we heap upon our bodies is often so overwhelming, it's a wonder the body functions at all.

We read and hear a lot about the impact of toxic exposure in our environment. And more and more frequently we hear about the influence that negative thinking can have on our health and well-being.

Yet, we rarely hear mentioned the toll our negative thoughts toward our body impacts its ability to function, or how these thoughts affect our self-esteem and overall well-being.

Our bodies reflect the essence of our humanness. It is time to make peace with your body.

The Fall In Love (FIL) Body Program & How It Began

A while back I had an experience that transformed my life—and my thoughts and feelings about my body—forever. *The FIL Body Program* is the result of that experience. I am excited to present *Fall in Love (FIL)* because I believe it can benefit you by transforming your life as well.

My body did change as a result of my new perspective; however, most importantly, something in me shifted. Life would never be quite the same. I inadvertently discovered this process as the result of a personal experience which led me to a profound discovery.

> **In a nutshell, my sometimes boyfriend told me he was no longer attracted to me because of my weight gain! I immediately was tempted to dust off my treadmill and hop on. Get back on track. I had been there before. But at that moment, something happened. I knew I had to find another way, a way that was more self-loving.**

I had gained about 25 pounds over that year. While he acknowledged that it might seem shallow, he said he believed it was important to "put up a struggle" to maintain our bodies.

Furthermore, he voiced his concern that if I consistently gained 20 pounds a year I would become quite large. I laugh when I imagine this part of it now—I actually find it to be rather humorous. In retrospect I can have a sense of humor about it, but at the time it was a big *ouch*.

Immediately feelings of humiliation, then hurt and anger, arose in me. My urge to jump on the treadmill wasn't related to him. It wasn't to try to get him back. Rather, *it was to squelch the feeling of shame that welled up in me about my body.* Maybe some of you can relate.

I had been through this cycle before. I knew how to "get in shape," exercise, eat healthier food, and take care of myself—I know that merry-go-round well.

While I am not saying this approach cannot "work" on some level, something in me knew that *I needed to find another way, that there was another perspective I could take, another approach, that would address my body and my relationship to myself on a whole new level. A level that I now know creates more lasting, more profound, and more joyful change.*

But at the time, I did not have a roadmap to guide me.

Although I had the urge to jump on my treadmill and make a monumental effort to make my body more appealing, I resisted. *Something indefinable took over and stopped me. I became still.* In that stillness, I experienced an "aha moment" and made a decision right then that changed my life. *I realized this was not about him, it was about my relationship with me.*

In resisting the urge to jump on the treadmill, both literally and physically, I found another path, a path that has brought me to a place of greater joy and true appreciation for my body—and for life. I can now say I deeply appreciate my body and all it does for me daily.

> **I decided not to take specific actions like dieting and exercising. Rather, I committed to falling in love with my body as it was right then in that moment. Loving my**

> **body not the way I wished it was or imagined it to be, but rather to appreciate what it gave to me now.**
>
> **Suddenly, in a flash, I realized my body is what allowed me to be here in this life, that I wouldn't exist without my body. A couple simple techniques I developed to re-frame how I viewed my body changed my life, and I believe it has the ability to transform yours.**

In the following weeks I developed a process that culminated in deeply altering, on a core level, how I experienced my body and how I felt towards it. I could never again treat it with disregard and disdain.

> **I did not know at the time that I would create a model for myself that might benefit others. But *I instinctively knew that the "old paradigm"—the way we as women have been trained to think about and treat our bodies—would not help or heal me.***

At the moment, I didn't realize how profound the change would be. *I just realized I needed to find a different way.* I needed to not get on the treadmill—a shame-based response—at least in that moment. As I resisted that urge, I discovered another path and learned that healing is possible, the kind of healing that we can relax into.

A Message For You

Let's go back to my experience for a moment because there is a message here for you. It's an important piece to understand.

Had I stayed in a state of focusing on my boyfriend by blaming or criticizing him, or had I given in to the urge to take action by dieting and exercise, nothing would have really changed. Nothing would be different. *Something had to change in me and the same is true for you.*

Strange as it may sound, I am grateful for that experience. It brought me to a whole new level of awareness and greater joy. More accurately, I feel I experienced a "calling" of sorts at that moment, and by following it I have become more integrated in relation to my body and my life. Best of all, I can help other women feel better about their bodies. And that is where you come in.

Let's talk briefly about my initial reaction of anger toward the bearer of the message. Anger can be valuable and informative. It can let us know that we're being treated in a manner we don't like, or that we don't feel good about a situation. Anger can prompt us to take action or make a change in our lives by leaving a situation that's not good for us.

Relative to my experience, it is understandable that anger would arise. I felt hurt—and anger is often the first response to feeling hurt. *Anger feels more empowering, less vulnerable than hurt.*

It was clear that I could get lots of support from others about what a jerk this person must be. How could he say something like that to me? He was right—he is shallow . . . blah blah blah. We all know the routine, "the story". We hear these stories every day in one form or another, and perhaps we even tell these stories ourselves once in a while . . . or maybe even frequently.

The truth is, though, these stories we tell ourselves are not empowering us. They turn us into victims and martyrs, and not only are the stories false, they do not make for a very enjoyable life. When feelings of hurt, anger, or resentment arise, it is important to allow ourselves to feel them for a time, but then it's just as necessary to *move on.*

If we stay stuck in the stories of how we were wronged, we go nowhere but down and don't create the life we deserve. We need to learn how to

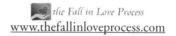

move through these emotions and then change our focus to something more life-affirming and empowering.

Blaming others disempowers you, and positive change cannot occur in a state of disempowerment. This is not to say that we're not impacted by others—of course we are. But we do not have to be controlled by them. Our sense of self does not need to be destroyed by others. If it can be, we're in trouble. We need never give someone that kind of power over us.

Empowerment comes from the inside, in knowing that you can connect with your own life in a way that allows you to experience all the joy and love you choose. Love and joy are **always** available to you. To believe that another person can take that away is a false perception—one that takes your personal power away.

Relationships are meaningful and significant in our lives. They matter. But our sense of self-worth must be built on something more than what a particular person thinks or feels about us, or we are on very shaky ground. Real self-worth is built from the inside out, not from the outside in. Otherwise you are dependent on others for your sense of self, and if you lose their approval your self-esteem plummets. Life is not fun in this state.

On that day, when I felt a stirring in a different direction, I believe it was toward a greater connection with the core of myself. I instinctively knew I needed to find another way, a way that embraced love for my body and self-love. Love for my body was a new concept. Maybe it is for you too. Yet, we cannot deeply love ourselves if we don't love our body.

Everything changes in relation to your body when you fall in love with it. You feel better about yourself. You are in greater balance. Your body can then become your friend and will respond to love with a greater sense of well-being. Just as you respond and blossom in receiving love, so does your body. You deserve to *Fall In Love*.

A Note To Men:

If you are a male who experiences negative thoughts and feelings about your body, this program can help you as well. *FIL* is focused upon women because generally women have more issues about their bodies. However, it's not my intention that it be exclusive to women.

The focus of the book has been on women because there has been tremendous pressure placed upon women regarding their bodies. Often, women come to believe that their entire value as a woman rests upon the physical appearance of their bodies.

Yet, there are men who may feel disempowered toward their bodies as well. In fact, several men have approached me to let me know they need help with negative feelings about their bodies. If this is you, feel free to participate. It would be great to have you.

CHAPTER ONE

Women & Their Bodies:
A Silent Epidemic Of Suffering

Stop it. Your body can hear everything you're saying.
—L.M. A FIL Student

When you betray yourself you are saying to yourself that you are no different from the people who hurt you.
-Caroline Myss

H ave you ever felt anxious, insecure, embarrassed, ashamed, or inadequate about your body? *Women suffer over their bodies.* Chances are that includes you.

Our suffering and sense of inadequacy as women is so commonplace that it is barely noticed. In fact, feeling bad about our bodies is so typical it is viewed as "normal". Is it normal to be this uptight about the body that gives us life? The suffering we women experience over our bodies is harming us.

We live in a time and culture in which criticizing our bodies has reached epidemic proportions. This is so common that we rarely question or challenge this negativity.

If "normal" is defined as what the majority adopts, then this mindset has become "the norm". Yet, *when the norm becomes destructive to one's well-being, it must be challenged and changed.*

Unfortunately, it is not a positive state that most of us are experiencing about our bodies. If this were the case we wouldn't be feeling the degree of anxiety, shame, and disappointment that is so typical for women relative to their bodies. We need healing.

This alienation from our bodies is pervasive, the consequences often sad, sometimes tragic. We cannot escape our bodies, for after all we're carrying them around with us (or rather our body is carrying us around) every single moment of our lives.

Our most intimate relationship is with our body, for it never leaves us for a single moment. It is with us always. There is nothing that is more intimate to our lives.

We, as women, have become so accustomed to not feeling good about our bodies—so used to criticizing them—that we don't even recognize what we're doing. *It is as if we're on automatic pilot.*

Women have accepted beliefs about their bodies for a very long time that are causing them to suffer. It doesn't have to be this way. *The time has come for it to change.*

The current status quo is all about the quest for the perfect body. *A quest that can never be fulfilled.* Something is drastically amiss when we can look in the mirror at an emaciated body and see it as fat. *This demonstrates how misled we can become by the current body paradigm* that teaches us our bodies aren't adequate.

Although many of us are not in this situation, we still are part of the epidemic and are being hurt by adopting beliefs about our bodies that are harmful.

Have you criticized specific parts of your body? For example, maybe you do not like your nose, your hair, your eyes, your breasts, or your hips. There is no end to the list.

Have you ever stopped yourself from attending an event or going somewhere (like the beach, a party, a date) because you felt too fat or thought you didn't look good enough?

Do you over exercise and feel anxious if you have to miss a workout? Are you fearful that even though your body looks "good" now, you may lose it at some point, so you have to work very hard to keep your "good" body?

Have you worried about what others think of your body? Do you spend an inordinate amount of time maintaining your body and/or appearance? Are you anxious about your body aging?

If you answered yes to any of these questions, chances are you have embraced the current body paradigm and your life is out of balance.

You are suffering deep down inside and no amount of diet, exercise, beauty products, or cosmetic procedures will "cure" the pain you're experiencing. The pain you have felt for so long you may not even realize you are feeling it.

It is similar to the feeling women have when they are alone outside at night. We have become so accustomed to the danger of being out alone that we take it for granted and do not allow ourselves to feel that we're living under siege. We somehow adapt. We stuff our feelings down and press forward, preferring not to talk about it, pretending it does not exist.

We do this with our negativity toward our bodies as well, except at a certain point it is self-imposed. It is not that we don't talk a lot about its shortcomings. Rather, we ignore the fact that we are hurting ourselves in the process.

I want to ask you a question relative to your self-criticism and feelings of inadequacy and anxiety over your body: *What has been the cost to you in terms of your overall well-being?* Now, imagine the cost if you continue in this way for the rest of your life.

Self-loathing in the form of criticizing our bodies is rampant; it is an out-of-control epidemic that goes on and on. We need to first become aware of and then stop doing this to ourselves.

Perhaps most amazing is that women of all sizes feel inadequate about their bodies. *This silent epidemic of suffering that women endure is not reserved for a certain body type. No woman is immune.*

Women in general feel anxious and critical of their bodies. *Women are trapped in a cycle of self-criticism that keeps them disconnected from the true nature of their bodies and themselves.* We are disempowering ourselves.

As I provide a few examples of the toll this epidemic takes upon women, you will see what I am talking about. Reflect upon the things you and your girlfriends say about your own bodies. Listen to conversations you hear when you are out in public and what women are saying about their bodies. You do not have to be out and about for any length of time before you hear women saying negative things about their bodies.

Consider the number of women and young girls who suffer from eating disorders. You might have noticed that eating disorders have increased greatly in our culture, approaching epidemic numbers.

Unfortunately, younger and younger girls are developing eating disorders. What a legacy to leave our daughters.

Let's take a look at the current body paradigm that women have embraced, often unknowingly, that keeps them feeling bad about their bodies.

The Current Body Paradigm That Keeps You Insecure & Anxious

A paradigm is a way of viewing a particular thing—or a worldview. A paradigm shift is a change from one way of thinking about something to another way of viewing it. A paradigm shift implies a radical transformation in our worldview or underlying belief system.

It is easy to recognize the current self-defeating body paradigm; that is, the status quo way of viewing our bodies. The current paradigm consists of all the beliefs we have picked up along the way that tell us our bodies are not good enough as they are.

The current paradigm implies that your value as a woman is all about your body. It has you questioning every aspect of your looks and body, and finding numerous criticisms. The current paradigm represents the beliefs we as women embrace that keep us in a cycle of feeling ashamed and inadequate about our bodies. The beliefs that keep us jumping on the treadmill and dieting.

This outdated current paradigm has you comparing yourself to other women, and competing with them. It has you spending inordinate amounts of time in front of a mirror. The current paradigm has you exercising frantically, worrying, and overly concerned with the normal aging process—something we will do anything to avoid!

Of course, the current body paradigm boiled down to its essence translates to, "You are not good enough as you are." Period. Yet, you'll likely do many things to try to meet what you perceive to be the current standard in relation to your body and how you look.

Being obsessed by your body and how you look hurts you and causes you to lose the person who you are really meant to be, if you were not downright neurotic about your body (do not feel alone, remember this is an epidemic).

Drinking the kool-aid

I call adopting the current paradigm (think: status quo beliefs about our bodies) with blind acceptance and without questioning *drinking the kool-aid.* You may have heard about the kool-aid.

Drinking the kool-aid means swallowing hook, line, and sinker all we have been taught and told about our bodies that keeps us not liking them, to put it mildly. When we drink the kool-aid, we betray ourselves.

It is time to stop drinking the kool-aid. Really, it's irrational if the truth be told. And you may have heard, the kool-aid is not good for you.

The basic assumption of the current paradigm is that your body needs significant improvement—always! The status quo body paradigm = feeling alienated and bad about your body. **You will never be adequate in the current body paradigm.**

Read this last statement again. You will never feel adequate while under the spell of the current paradigm. Ponder the implications. Do you realize how vulnerable you are to being manipulated when you embrace the current paradigm? It is time to get mad about this—and then get motivated!

The current paradigm keeps you feeling anxious and insecure about your body. It does not feel good, yet it is familiar. Like a dysfunctional relationship.

How often do you hear women speak well of their bodies? How often do you hear women complain about and criticize their bodies? How often do you speak well about your body? How often do you criticize your body?

By now you probably understand what I mean when I say women are suffering from a silent epidemic. On second thought, it is not that silent! *The silent aspect is that it is not being acknowledged or addressed for what it is—harmful.*

You can barely leave your house without hearing women's endless negative chatter about how unacceptable or imperfect their bodies are. You hear it in the cafes, the gym, the beauty shop, the clothing store, and especially in the dressing room. Can you believe some of the mirrors they have in those rooms? It's enough to make you shudder. That's what I'm talkin' about.

The simple reality is that under *the current paradigm your body will never be good enough.* Now, that leaves you in a bind. *You will continue to work hard to meet a standard that is impossible to meet. And even if you did, it would not bring you the happiness you imagined it would.* A losing proposition all the way around.

> **The belief that you need to constantly strive for the perfect body occurs regardless of your body type.** *It does not matter whether you are thin, overweight, or "just right".*
>
> **The message is the same: You will *never* be adequate. This message is ingrained in us. Not all that pleasant, wouldn't you agree? And we are our own worst critics. Why? Because *we have bought into the current paradigm and are operating on automatic pilot.***

In the current outdated paradigm it is likely you have accepted—and perpetuated, yes ladies you heard me correctly—beliefs about your body that prevent you from feeling really good about yourself on a core level. It's understandable. We have picked up on this message all our lives.

In addition to our personal feelings and beliefs about our bodies, there are collective perceptions that impact how we view our bodies. These are societal views. In fact, our personal beliefs and feelings usually arise from collective perceptions and this is how the current paradigm evolved. *Yet, the reasons why are not as important as knowing how to change it.*

If you pay attention to conversations around you, movies, and advertising, you will recognize that there are common perceptions within the collective consciousness about women and their bodies. The emphasis on having to look a certain way has created an industry where billions of dollars are made by creating products and procedures which are geared toward helping you look better and feel better about your body.

Of course, in order to be incredibly successful in selling products and procedures, one needs to create a sense of insecurity in a woman about her body. Otherwise, she would not become the great customer they desire. A lack has to be perceived or the products or procedures will not be purchased. And you may have noticed, cosmetic procedures are becoming commonplace.

I have even seen advertisements for vaginal cosmetic surgery. Have we gone mad? Now, I get it that if a woman has a medical condition, this may be necessary, but tell me honestly . . . are we actually paying to have our vaginas manipulated while women in some parts of the world are trying to gain the right to not have their genitals mutilated. Ironic. Where will the craziness end?

The thing about this is that when our feelings and beliefs are coming from outside us rather than inside we are in a precarious position. Self-esteem is generated from the inside out, not the outside in.

If our sense of value as a person comes from the outside, we allow others to define us rather than defining ourselves. We become very vulnerable to manipulation. Sometimes there are ulterior motives. **The beauty industry is capitalizing on your insecurity.**

In considering the impact the current paradigm has upon you, think about this: Is there anything other than your body you spend every single second of your life with? The answer is obvious, yet we don't think about this and even less so the impact your negativity has upon your body.

That means you're being nasty and negative to your only constant companion and you're doing it without awareness.

> *Would you talk about your friends the way you talk about your body? If not, why not and why do you continue to talk about your body in such a way? I'll answer that for you—habit.*

Have you ever wondered about the toll this takes on your psyche and spirit, not to mention your health and self-esteem? To disregard an aspect of yourself that is central to who you are. Your negative feelings about your body is not good for your overall well-being and it is not making for the best life ever.

The nature of the current body paradigm happens to be that you end up feeling anxious, inadequate, and ashamed about your body. *Shame by its nature keeps you disempowered.*

Shame and disempowerment makes you *controllable.* You will jump through more and more hoops to feel "good enough" about yourself, whether it is by buying more and more products or doing anything that makes itself available to you that promises you'll be acceptable and beautiful.

9

The greater your shame, the lower your self-esteem. The less worthy you feel, the more others can control you. You lose your power. The power that enables you to value and take care of yourself. Unwittingly, you betray yourself in the process.

The reasons why we have evolved such negative feelings about our bodies are many and varied, but they do not really matter in the end. What matters is that the current body paradigm has gone on way too long and it is not going to disappear on its own.

The time to change is now and you have the power to change it. In fact, only you can. Learning how to love your body will require a willingness to step out of the current paradigm.

Sadly, women up to this point have not had a different model to embrace. Therefore, the silent epidemic of suffering has continued. Enter the beauty industry.

The Beauty Industry—The Billion Dollar Machine That Plays You Like A Puppet On A String

Understand this: **The beauty industry makes billions of dollars by convincing you that you are not adequate as you are.**

You need a variety of expensive products and procedures to make you more acceptable—and yet, there's no end to jumping through the hoops once you begin. There is no way out because you will *never* measure up while operating under the current paradigm. But by god, you will give it your all trying.

The industry is INVESTED in you! But the question is, what is the nature of the investment?

I'll give you a big hint:

> **If you can be manipulated to feel that you are inadequate as you are now, you are a vast reservoir of financial gain for the beauty industry. Yet, the truth is, *you can never purchase enough products or have enough procedures to bring you the comfort to feel that once and for all you are adequate.***

Why? Because a feeling of adequacy and self-worth are an inside job! I repeat this for it's worth getting it into your noggin'—*your sense of well-being and the value you place on yourself is an inside job.* No one and nothing outside yourself can make you feel good about yourself. Now, that is a secret you will never learn from the beauty industry.

This is actually great news for it means *you* and you alone have the *power* to change how you feel. But first you need to question the current outdated paradigm *if you want to feel better about your body—and yourself!*

Adopting the current body paradigm for so long means you've been on automatic pilot about your body. You have not questioned. You are unknowingly committed to the status quo. You're feeding the beast!

Be honest with yourself: *Have you unknowingly adopted the current body paradigm that keeps you* feeling anxious and insecure about your body? If so, you probably experience a deep down feeling that your body is not good enough and fear that it will never be. That feeling makes you want to not look in a mirror or turn all the lights out when you make love. Worse yet, maybe to not make love at all.

This anxiety and shame is reflected by the voice inside your head that tells you maybe you shouldn't go to the party or beach because you think your butt is too big. Do not even give your power away by asking your boyfriend or husband. Never ask again. Just don't.

There are reasons why we as women have endorsed beliefs about ourselves that have kept us feeling ashamed and inadequate about our bodies. For decades our self-worth has been tied to how attractive our bodies are.

Unfortunately, one of the highest costs is that we go to extremes to have a great body and most of us still do not feel good about our bodies. *No matter how many products you buy, you still worry that you don't look good. Even if your body looks okay now, it could betray you at any time.* You are on edge.

Remember ladies, these feelings are not confined to overweight women. Thin women suffer too. Maybe you know someone who has an amazing body by cultural standards, yet if you ask her how she feels about her body, she is in a turmoil inside. In fact, this woman often feels tremendous anxiety about her body.

Regardless of how or why things are as they are, as a woman there is something that is very important for you to recognize:

> **You do not have to accept feeling anxious, ashamed, and bad about your body as a way of life. Nobody has a gun to your head.**

Your first step toward change is taking a good square look at what is. *Take a look at all the ways you have been adopting the current body paradigm.* If you decide you do not like what is, determine to make a change.

Not A Campaign Against Beauty

I'm Not Saying Be Ugly

*L*earning to value your body is not about being unattractive or not caring about how you look. It's about creating balance in your life.

The point is not that everyone should just let it all hang out with no thought of looking good or taking care of themselves. Come on, let's get real! That is not the point at all.

Coming to appreciate your body is *not* about being against anything. Rather it is about embracing your body in a way you have probably never done. You have the power over your own life. In order to exercise your power though, you need to get real about the current reality.

Learning a new way to view your body that is more life-affirming is about *taking yourself off auto-pilot* and learning *a new way of thinking about your body* that will help *free* you from anxiety and shame and **empower you to be the woman that deep down you know you are capable of being.** It is not against beauty, it is about *balancing your life*.

There is nothing wrong with purchasing beauty products and wanting to look lovely. What makes it truly fun, though, is when we do this from a place of feeling good about our body rather than from a desperate and anxious attempt to make it different because we dislike it—and ourselves.

You can come into greater alignment and balance in your life, learning to appreciate your body in a new way and embracing other important aspects of yourself rather than over-focusing upon your body.

You can be attractive *and* love your body.

Why Do I Need To Change?

*Y*ou need to unlearn the kool-aid drinking syndrome! It is important to examine the current body paradigm, understand the harm it causes you, and make a different, more life-affirming choice. You need to create a new more empowered way of thinking and feeling about your body.

By learning a few simple tools, processes, concepts, and powerful "exercises" you can reframe your whole concept of your body and develop a new appreciation for it.

The exercises are designed to incorporate these good feelings about your body into your core, in such a way that you will never again be able to dislike or put down your body without becoming keenly aware of what you are doing. At that point, you can get back on track easily before you have a train wreck.

In essence, *you need to* change how you think and feel about your body.

> *The whole point is for you to recognize that disliking your body is not a functional, emotionally happy way to live, and it doesn't have to be this way. The status quo does not equal happy. You pay a high price for embracing beliefs that hurt you, buying into the current paradigm wholeheartedly without questioning.*

Decades slip by and *we women are still trapped in a cycle of anxiety, criticism, and disconnection from our bodies.* Why?

The fact that women's negativity toward their bodies is a rampant epidemic has probably led you to accept feeling bad about your body as normal. It is just the way it is, you tell yourself.

That is what happens when we do not even recognize there is an epidemic. We become our own worst enemies. Out of sight, out of mind. *We stay blinded and in denial about reality.* This is a real problem because we cannot begin to change something of which we are unaware.

The reality is obvious to anyone who chooses to take a look. *How is it we keep missing the obvious and perpetuating the epidemic?* We as women are so conditioned in the current paradigm that, although painful, it feels normal. If normal is average, then it is. *Does that make it good?*

I know several women who are so obsessed about their bodies that it seriously negatively impacts the quality of their relationships and their lives. Are you one of those women?

Because we are so accustomed to criticizing our bodies we do not really consider there may be another way or that there's anything "abnormal" about it. After all, everywhere we turn we hear and see women doing the same thing—saying terrible things about their bodies—and we participate. *It's the norm.*

But I have a couple questions for you to ask yourself:

- *Does the current body paradigm help you feel good about yourself?*
- *Does it improve your self-esteem or diminish you?*

I cannot imagine the body is happy about all the bad press it's receiving from the women it provides a house for.

Even the medical profession recognizes that our thoughts and emotions impact our physical health, as well as our emotional well-being. Yet, *we rarely hear this applied to how we think, talk, and feel about our own bodies.*

We as women have largely "swallowed" whole the current paradigm about our bodies.

The current paradigm:

- Keeps you *trapped in your own insecurities and anxieties*
- Creates *emotional discomfort and pain in your life*
- Keeps you *disempowered and feeling inadequate*
- It is just *not fun*

If any of the following applies to you, the FIL Body Program can be of benefit:

Diet and exercise programs have failed

You are unhappy about your body

You feel anxious, inadequate, or ashamed of your body

You have limited your activities over embarrassment about your body

You are tired of feeling bad about your body

You are obsessed with diet and exercise

You feel okay about your body now but feel compelled to work hard to maintain it

You are afraid of aging and what it will do to your body

You want to learn how to befriend your body

You are open to a new perspective that might help you feel a whole lot better

You want to become more empowered

You are willing to embrace the thought of radical transformation

You are willing to put in the effort that change requires

You want to be part of a community of women who are learning to fall in love

Remember, **women of all body types have plugged into the current body paradigm that is harmful—it is NOT only about weight.**

It takes *courage* to change. The truth is *most people are willing to live within the status quo. The cutting edge isn't crowded.*

Most of us are comfortable operating within the current body paradigm, even though it is painful. We may be stuck and unhappy, but it is familiar and we may not recognize the toll it's taking on our lives. That is why I call it the silent epidemic. We have adapted to the pain. We do not want to make the effort to participate in a program of change. I have been there myself more than once in my life and I'm sure I'll visit there again. *Here is the point; although we may visit the lazy place from time to time, we don't have to live there!*

I get it. Sometimes we have to experience enough pain that we realize it is less painful to act than to continue down the same road.

Adopting the current body paradigm implies that your self-worth is being generated from the outside in. A sense of worth you gain from the outside in (that is, being admired by others) while it feels good, will never be enough in itself. You need to feel your self-worth in the core of your being and that experience does not come from others. A true sense of self-worth comes from inside yourself.

Depending upon others for your sense of adequacy places you at the mercy of someone else. It is like an earthquake waiting to happen. It makes your happiness and well-being dependent upon what others think and how others perceive you. *It weakens you and makes you vulnerable and controllable. You lose yourself.* That is what happens when you plug into the current body paradigm.

In order to love your body, you need to learn how to begin, moment by moment, to appreciate and marvel at this incredible body you have been given that carries you through life.

While it may seem impossible to you now, at some point your appreciation for your body will become second nature.

In a way it's like re-programming the software in a computer. You simply need to remove the old self-defeating software and add the new uplifting program (don't worry it's not brainwashing, it is adding beliefs that help you love yourself more).

> **Women, it is time to rattle the cage the current paradigm has you in. Better yet, it is time to break out of it. The belief that your body is not good enough has a logical conclusion. The conclusion is that you are not good enough as a woman.**

The time has come for women to question the status quo. The status quo is the beliefs we have "swallowed" for decades that keep us feeling bad about our body—and therefore ourselves. *It has to do with over-identifying with the body in a way that is disempowering and to the point of diminishing other aspects of ourselves and our lives.*

Think about it. Your body is the core of you. If your body is not good enough, you are not good enough. It is crazy-making, really, to not appreciate the vehicle that gives you life.

Ladies, let's face it, regardless of how this all began, at this point we are disempowering ourselves. We have lost our balance and we can regain it. First, we need to own it and then we need guidance on how to change it.

The Body Program provides that guidance.

Do not despair over the current state of affairs. *I would not be bringing this up if I didn't believe there's a way through to the other side.* We can change what we have learned and begin anew with a fresh outlook.

If you are out of balance regarding how you feel about your body, it is not going to magically correct itself, but it can get better. The first step is recognizing the problem.

What Makes The Fall In Love Body Program Unique?

*T*he *Body Program* is different from other body programs.

> *Falling In Love* is a *unique* process that provides a model to deeply change your feelings about your body so that you can feel better about it—and your life. The time has come for women to embrace a new paradigm, a new way of viewing our bodies that is more affirming and empowered, more loving.

*This process is **not** about teaching you to stand in front of the mirror and say "I love you" to jutting hips or various body parts you aren't pleased with! Truly, do you think your mind or hips believe that?* That is kind of like looking at a big pimple on your face and saying over and over how much you love it.

Really? I hate to be the bearer of bad tidings, but do not count on these kinds of affirmations to be effective. In order for change to occur, you must *feel* it, not just say affirmations that come from the mind alone.

In order to love your body *the way you think and feel about your body must change. Reframing* is a technique you will learn that will change how you focus when you think about your body. This is an entirely different way of approaching things. You need to focus upon your body in a new way.

The Body Program is **not** about diet and exercise. We have plenty of that sort of information out there. While it is important to eat well and take care of our bodies, **there is a missing link that is a main reason, from my perspective, that diets and exercise tend to fail**.

Ask yourself this question: **If you dislike something are you inclined to want to take good care of it?** The answer is obvious. In order to treat your body well, you *first* have to *value* it.

Changing how we feel about our bodies necessitates a shift from the inside out. *Exercise programs and dieting promote change from the outside in.* Although they may be beneficial, the changes we experience are often short-lived and do not last. Much to our dismay, diet and exercise often do not work in the long run, and we will take a closer look at why this is later.

At the moment, suffice it to say **diet and exercise do not heal the shame, anxiety, and pain that you feel and they do not help you love your body. Self-love is the missing aspect. Therefore, the whole foundation for healing and change is not present.**

In order to be lasting, change needs to occur inside ourselves and that change will then be reflected in our outer world. If we don't like our bodies, we are not really inspired because we do not really value them. As you learn to actually love your body, you become inspired to want to be good to it. You value your body in a new way.

A key element of *The Body Program* is reframing (changing) your perspective in a way that enables you to begin viewing your body in a whole different light. *It has everything to do with where you place your focus.*

Shifting your focus makes all the difference in the way you think and feel about your body by helping you change from looking at what you don't like to deeply experiencing what you love and appreciate.

How we focus, what we pay attention to, is incredibly significant. We tend to get what we focus upon and how and what we focus on largely determines the course of our lives.

For most women, the focus toward our bodies has been on what we do not like. That must change if we want to feel better about our bodies.

Remember, *FIL* is not a weight loss program. Although weight loss may be a result, the primary focus is on falling in love with your body. Many benefits will be realized through this process.

Ironically, many women who fit the standard ideal are in tremendous emotional pain and anxious about their bodies as well. I have known many women who by society's standard are absolutely beautiful and yet they still feel inadequate and empty inside. Many of these women exercise frantically and often women who look like models experience a tremendous sense of inadequacy and become obsessed about their bodies. Consequently, *FIL* is for all body types.

In attempting to be "perfect" we deprive ourselves of the basic pleasures, such as the ability to enjoy a lovely meal without anxiety and worry. *Many women experience tremendous anxiety every time they go to eat or even think about eating.*

While this may be typical, it is not inherent to who we are as human beings. This is a learned behavior that's a result of believing in the current paradigm. We need a different viewpoint in order to change this.

It pains me to hear women talk about their bodies with such negativity. Take a look around—and listen. I know that you know what I am talking about.

While some men experience deeply painful body issues as well, most men are not obsessed by it. They do not experience the same sort of pressure, as their self-worth is usually not as identified through their looks and bodies. It is noteworthy, however, that it seems more men are developing these issues and a market has developed to exploit their increased insecurities relative to their bodies.

Since many women suffer over their bodies even when they are an ideal weight, it is important to offer assistance to women of all sizes and shapes. *The FIL Body Program* is not about weight, it is about instilling self-worth by adopting a whole new perspective.

We all recognize that there is a multi-million dollar industry helping to ensure that we do *not* feel good enough about ourselves, so that we will purchase lots of beauty and diet products—and we do.

There is nothing "wrong" with buying beauty products and wanting to look lovely, but when we become obsessed and jump on a merry-go-round that leads to diets, failures, and repeated plunging of our self-esteem, we suffer. We need to come into balance and heal.

This process is designed to help you step off that merry-go-round and become empowered to love your body—and in the process yourself. Your focus will shift to the tremendous benefits your body affords you—like being alive!

The Key To Why Diets & Exercise Fail

E xercise and diets may be beneficial at times; however, more often than not they fail in the long run.

> *How many times have you been on the diet/exercise merry-go-round? How is it working for you? Even if you've been successful with dieting and exercise, do you feel secure about your body or are you anxious and obsessed about it?*

Imagine for a moment you're wanting to build a house. What do you think would happen if you didn't know that in order to build a house it needs a foundation? How successful would you be?

Now, think about how you feel about your body. Unless you begin from a place of loving and appreciating your body, how successful do you think "diet" and exercise will be? The answer is not very and that is because *if you don't like your body, you won't value it.*

This is extremely significant. Think about the things you value in your life and the things you don't. *Which do you want to take care of? The value you place on something says everything about how you treat it.*

Diets and exercise fail because unless you love and value your body, *you tend to force yourself* to diet and exercise. If you're forcing action, rather than inspired to take action it does not tend to last in the long run.

Equally important, diets and exercise fail to address the root of the issue—your lack of love and appreciation for your body.

I know what you are probably thinking and it is likely something you've been telling yourself all your life. **I will love my body when it is better, when it looks the way I want it to look.**

How well is that working for you so far? It does not work because it's putting the cart before the horse. It may not make sense to you rationally, but trust me on this, it is not how things work.

Maybe you have heard about the law of attraction: "That which is like unto itself is drawn?" You must love your body first. Otherwise, it is like trying to attract money by constantly focusing on the lack of it. It does not work.

Love your body first and the rest will fall into place.

Women's Relationship With Food

I n order to help you understand the depth of the pain women suffer over their bodies we need to talk a bit more about women and their relationship with food.

Let's start with the fact that food is what sustains you, fuels your body, and keeps you alive. Delicious food can be a source of great joy to the palate. Food is a way that we commune and socialize with friends and loved ones.

Yet, for many women *the way food is perceived has become tremendously distorted. Somehow, what sustains us has become the enemy and something we are terribly frightened of.*

I will always remember the women in one of my groups for an intensive inpatient program for eating disorders. They were a wonderful and likable group of young women, struggling heroically with their disorders. It was stunning to watch their relationship with food.

As you can imagine, when food is the addiction, eating in the cafeteria is a major affair that brings up intense anxiety. Each day when the women came to group they would admit their obsession with what they ate and what other women in the group ate. They could name what the others had eaten, as well as themselves and focused upon this in great detail. Women talked about hoarding and hiding food in their rooms, ashamed to eat publicly.

Next came the obsession with exercising daily, often to an extreme. This was another topic discussed at great length.

What struck me most profoundly was that these women truly were awesome and yet the degree of their anxiety and suffering was intense.

They were in tremendous pain. Their focus on food, exercise, and their bodies consumed them. *There was no room to focus upon or enjoy other areas of life.* A sense of balance had been lost.

Not all of us suffer to this extent, but for many there is anxiety around food and a lack of balance in relationship to it.

What is your relationship with food? Do you feel comfortable with the food you put in your mouth or do you eat with a feeling of "I shouldn't be eating this" as you pop the food in your mouth and swallow.

Doing this is not promoting emotional health or even physical well-being. A healthy perspective is to be congruent in your thought and action. Make peace with the food you eat before you put it in your mouth and swallow it.

> **Healing your relationship with food involves making peace with everything you place in your mouth. Healing your relationship with exercise means that you are not frantically exercising. Rather you are exercising to a reasonable degree.**
>
> **The same can be said for purchasing and using beauty products, the time we spend on our looks, and having cosmetic procedures.**
>
> **It's about balance.**

The Real Reason You Want A "Perfect" Body

Perhaps one of the saddest aspects of women working so hard at trying to have a perfect body is that we are not in touch with the real reason we're doing it. Coupled with the fact that we will not ever achieve the "perfect" body and therefore we are doomed to failure, there is another aspect that's even worse.

The real reason we want a great body (other than for good health) is that we feel we are not valuable or lovable if our bodies do not meet the standard that is expected. We are not really seeking the perfect body, we're seeking love and acceptance. The value we place on ourselves as women is all wrapped up in our bodies.

Another tragic consequence is that even when we do achieve an awesome body, we still feel anxious and worried.

These are the dilemmas the current paradigm has placed us in. These are the ways we betray ourselves, jumping through impossible hoops and not addressing the core issue—a desire to feel loved and valued.

Self-Betrayal & Empowered Choice

If you look back to the quotes at the beginning of this chapter you will notice they are about self-betrayal. By adopting the current paradigm of criticizing our bodies we are betraying ourselves. But *before you blame yourself, realize that you cannot change that which is outside your awareness.*

The beliefs we have adopted relative to the current paradigm are similar to a dynamic that often occurs during childhood. Many children are told certain negative things about themselves that they internalize and later play out as adults.

For example, if someone was told they were stupid as a child, they are likely to have a voice inside as an adult that tells them the same thing. This is what it means to internalize something of this nature. Initially we are told something about ourselves and later as adults we find that we play those same beliefs like tapes over and over in our mind. It is almost like it's been recorded in our brains.

The message could be anything. You might have been told you were selfish as a child and in adulthood find yourself thinking (the internal voice) that you are selfish anytime you want to place yourself first—or even consider yourself for that matter.

This common psychological experience we have, the internalization of negative things we're told as a child, is a habit we perpetuate and continue into our adulthood. An unconscious habit.

Internalizing these negative messages means that we end up as adults telling ourselves the same negative things someone else told us when we were young. *We become our own harshest critic.*

We have internalized the current paradigm beliefs about our bodies that we have learned all our lives.

Now that you are aware of the current paradigm and the harm it causes you, you can begin to question it and take command of your choices (that is, have more options). As you begin to become more empowered by expanding your options, you will start feeling better about yourself. At a certain point you are no longer willing to allow outside forces to define who you are and your value as a woman.

At this point, it becomes more difficult to betray yourself. Rather than focus upon how it came to be this way and blaming others, you will find yourself attending to how you can free yourself. For in the end, we realize it is we who diminish ourselves and we become unwilling to continue down that path.

We all have self-defeating thoughts, feelings, and emotions that arise. In itself, this isn't a problem. We are not here to become "perfect," for that will not happen, nor is it meant to. We are here to enjoy life. The problem is when we get stuck in self-defeating thoughts and emotions. Visiting these places is one thing, living there is another.

Here is how this applies to your body. You got the message early on that your body had to be "perfect" in order for you to be valuable and loved, and the dilemma is that no matter what you do, your body will never be good enough. This translates as you are not good enough. You internalized this message and now impose this devastating message upon yourself.

Every time you criticize your body, you are in essence betraying yourself. You are pitting yourself against yourself. You are disconnecting from the core of your being, your very existence.

As you begin to question the current paradigm and adopt a new way of thinking and feeling about your body, you will begin to feel better about yourself. You will no longer be willing to betray your body—or yourself.

Your body allows you to exist. How much better could it be?

Women Are In This Together

A gain, the belief that there is something "bad" about your body and your body is inadequate is not reserved for any particular body type. *Women of ALL body types suffer.*

Making other women into enemies is falling for the current outdated paradigm. If you feel envious of other women and resent them it shows how much pain you are in. Be gentle with yourself as you heal and recognize it comes from a feeling of inadequacy. As you come to love your body and yourself this feeling is likely to decrease significantly.

This whole business of thin-fat finger pointing must stop. As I said before, it is not about weight. Reach for the healing salve. You are not the only one in pain. Support your sisters and reach out for their support.

The failure to value our bodies crosses all boundaries: socioeconomic, race, education level, body type, and personality style.

In order to heal, it helps to enlist the support of and be supportive of other women. Besides, *life is enriched tremendously by befriending other women.*

Most women are to some degree anxious and suffering, having experienced years of emotional pain, shame, or anxiety, in relationship to their bodies. For many women, this cycle of self-hatred regarding their bodies lasts a lifetime.

Women are in crisis over their bodies. Don't judge other women because their bodies are different from yours.

When we are feeling anxiety and emotional pain in relation to our bodies, it can be irritating and upsetting to hear someone talk about how great our bodies are. As you begin to feel better about your body, these feelings will subside. Women need the support of one another in this process.

Change Does Happen

I want to point out something that will help you realize that change in your own life is not only possible, but probable.

Think back 5, 10, or 20 years. Do you recall habits, patterns, ways of thinking or behaving that have changed in your life? I would bet that you do. This is because we do learn and grow. Old habits and patterns do fall away.

As you reflect back, you will see that indeed you have grown. *You are not the person you were a decade ago.* Appreciate yourself for your personal growth and let it be an incentive to move forward.

It may be challenging at first, but stay with FIL until you reap the tremendous benefits of the program. I know that you may want to throw *FIL* down when you first hear about what a great opportunity you have being in this physical life and how amazing your body is and what it does for you. The degree of your wanting to do so is probably proportional to the amount of pain you are in.

Hang in there. Remember, this is the purpose of the process. If you felt your body was great and your best friend right now you would **not** be reading this book.

You can go back to *FIL* at any time. You may want to repeat it at times when you feel yourself slipping. There is no right or wrong way to utilize this information. I only ask that you include and in some manner incorporate the "core" of the program, specifically the written exercise.

Although you may sometimes slip back into old patterns, your primary response will become one of appreciation, perhaps even adulation. When you get off track, you will have the tools to put yourself back in a place of appreciation quickly.

Everyone responds differently to information, depending upon where they are in their lives. Some topics are more easily incorporated than others. Do not become discouraged. Your well-being can increase exponentially. What do you have to lose?

Incorporating this information into your life will allow you to improve other areas of your life, as well as creating positive feelings about your body. Increasing your feelings of self-worth and well-being changes the nature of your relationships with others. The better you feel about yourself and the greater your sense of well-being, the more likely it is that your relationships will improve as well as other areas of your life. In order for this to happen, though, you need to use the program.

I cannot make promises to you regarding change in your personal life, although I believe this program has the potential to make a significant difference. I can only present the tools to get you there and provide support to you in your own process. It is up to you to take responsibility for creating the life you desire. If you are willing to put forth just a small amount of effort the rewards can be tremendous.

A core belief that many people hold is that change has to be hard and we have to struggle in order to experience change. In reality, it does not have to be hard.

The joy of embracing a path of personal growth is in knowing that it is not a linear process. Once we have become aware or conscious in a certain area of our lives, we can never quite go back to or remain in old, outworn patterns that don't serve us any longer.

You know deep inside that you have knowledge that allows you to access a place of greater health and well-being. This knowledge calls you back to a place of greater freedom and joy.

"Inspiration and embracement" describes the path that we will travel. This program is not about forcing yourself to change. Rather, it is about embracing change. One is a frantic approach, one is relaxing into a sense of well-being and embracement.

Change does happen.

CHAPTER TWO

You & Your Body

Love is the best nourishment you can feed your cells.
—Dr. Bruce Lipton
Cell Biologist

Your Body Is Not Inferior—It Is Magnificent

The body is arguably the most complex and magnificent thing that exists on the face of the earth—and beyond.

It has been estimated that our bodies perform about 100,000 activities every second in order to keep us alive and functioning. We have over 100 trillion cells in our body, more than all the stars in the Milky Way Galaxy. Our bodies are made up of the stuff of the stars (Deepak Chopra).

A tremendous exhibit has been on display in several cities called "Bodies: The Exhibition." If you have the opportunity, I recommend you view it. You will come away with a new appreciation for your body—unless you're squeamish, in which case you may want to avoid it. The exhibit shows real-life bodies and you see every single body part, including the muscles, tendons, nervous system, and organs.

You are a physical being focused in a physical body and your body is remarkable. By your very nature, your self and your body are inextricably intertwined. They are inseparable. The body that houses you is magnificent. Your body gives you life and provides a foundation for the rest of your functions: mind, emotions, and spirit.

Your magnificent body is impacted by your beliefs.

Your Beliefs Impact Your Well-Being and Health

A remarkable biologist, Bruce H. Lipton, Ph.D. has made groundbreaking contributions in the area of how our beliefs impact us. Dr. Lipton has a background as a medical school professor and research scientist. He has written extensively about the biology of belief. His work as a cell biologist lends an invaluable perspective in this regard.

Discoveries that Lipton made through the course of his research led him to re-evaluate certain core assumptions. He made significant discoveries relative to how cells receive and process information.

Lipton demonstrated that **we are not only a product of and at the mercy of our genes.** Rather, according to Lipton, *the way that we interact with, respond to, and perceive our environment actually determines the biology of our cells.*

Dr. Lipton made the remarkable discovery that *our genes adapt to our beliefs!* This is a radical shift from our past perspective, which held that genes and DNA control our biology.

Instead, Dr. Lipton contends, our DNA is responding to signals from outside the cell, and specific to our purposes, *our cells respond to our thoughts.* The cells respond either negatively or positively, depending upon our focus, specifically to what we're thinking and perceiving. That is big!

Dr. Lipton's research has indicated that we are controlled by our perceptions. How we perceive and react to our environment depends upon how our brains interpret the environment. Perhaps Lipton's most astounding statement is contained in a video interview on You Tube on cell biology. He states that **"Belief can re-write your genes."**

Dr. Lipton tells us that "**Love is the best nourishment you can feed your cells.**" Do you see how much control you have over your own well-being?

Recognizing the significance of your relationship with your body and holding more loving thoughts enables your body to relax. You can begin to heal as you embrace it with love. Be gentle with your body.

Real healing takes place in a state of love. As Lipton points out, love is the best nourishment you can feed yourself. Healing occurs from a place of reverence and love, playfulness and fun. From this place, our bodies can rejoice and begin to function in a more healthful manner.

We can begin to feel significantly better—physically, emotionally, mentally, and spiritually—as we align with our bodies and become allies with it. It is a natural progression, the outcome of loving your body.

The bottom line is that loving your body can promote healing and well-being. Disliking your body creates discord inside of you. Change your feelings about your body and stack the odds in your favor when it comes to health and healing. *Your body is waiting for you to fall in love!*

The Placebo Effect

The placebo effect is fascinating, as it demonstrates how the simple *belief* that one has received medicine can promote a healing response even when the actual pill has no medicinal benefit whatsoever.

In experiments that include a placebo—that is, a substance, that has no benefit in curing the particular medical condition—the purpose is to compare the results of the placebo to that of the actual drug. Individuals do not know which they are getting, the placebo or the "real" drug.

The remarkable part is that people often respond positively to the placebo, improving, even though there is no therapeutic benefit in the substance (most often a sugar pill).

What are these individuals responding to? A belief!

These individuals are responding to the belief that the substance will be of benefit. In this regard, the placebo phenomenon has provided us with valuable information about the human mind and its powerful impact on what we experience.

Your Body Is Literally Having to Fight You To Stay Well

Your thoughts and beliefs impact your life. Since most of us do not feel good about our bodies, we are at an immediate disadvantage. We are already "feeding" our bodies' negativity on a daily basis and that impacts our cells and consequently our health.

Cells (and therefore bodies) do not function well on negativity. This is significant to recognize for your health and your life in general. Think for a moment of the impact of negative thinking on your body on a daily basis. Think about the impact over months, years, and a lifetime.

We hear a lot about the impact of negative thinking on our lives and health these days. Yet, in spite of women's negativity toward their bodies, little is noted about the impact this has upon our overall health and well-being.

How does it feel to your body when you heap insults upon it? How might your body feel if your thoughts of your body are deeply appreciative?

Can you see that it may be detrimental, these negative feelings we harbor toward our bodies? And how wonderful it might feel to feel positive emotions toward it.

You *are* your body, your body is you. Being dissatisfied with and criticizing your body is being dissatisfied with and criticizing yourself.

Is this life-affirming? What is the impact on our bodies, our health, when we care so little for the vehicle that carries us through our life? How can the body create the best health ever if we are so very alienated from it?

> **If we do not feel well physically it is difficult to function. Just as when we eat junk food we do not feel good, when we pour junky thoughts into our head daily about how terrible our bodies are, we don't feel good. I cannot imagine our body enjoys it either.**
>
> **Stop fighting your body's ability for wellness. Begin feeding your body the thoughts that will help heal your relationship to your best friend that carries you through this life. Allow your body to thrive by aligning with it.**

Your body! The magnificent vehicle that carries you through your entire life journey, every moment, every breath, every experience. This wonderful body that enables you to exist in the here and now! How can you not love your body when you look at it this way?

As you come to love your body, it can relax and not have to work so hard to stay well.

Choosing Empowered Beliefs

Becoming aware of your beliefs may be one of the best things you can do to improve your life. In addition to the benefit to your life in general, becoming aware of your beliefs may reveal more about what you experience regarding your body—and your relationship with your body—than any other single factor. In fact, your beliefs are largely responsible for what you create in every area of your life.

*A helpful approach is to focus up*on the beliefs you wish to embrace rather than those that aren't working. Still, it's helpful to gain an understanding of how your current beliefs about your body are impacting your life now. It is important to know so you can change those beliefs that interfere with your ability to have a great relationship with your body.

Your *self-talk* provides very important clues about how you feel towards your body. Self-talk is the thoughts that go through your mind that may remain unspoken. It is what you silently say to yourself, your internal messages that you are feeding yourself on a regular basis. Your self-talk is your thought diet. We tend to play the same "tapes" (thoughts) through our minds repeatedly unless we learn how to interrupt those thoughts and replace them with new ones.

To determine your beliefs about your body, pay attention to what you say to yourself and others about it. Notice the things you say about your body in your mind, to your friends, and to your family. Jot down the things you find yourself thinking (self-talk) and saying.

It is a fine line between exploring your limiting beliefs in order to create new ones and over-focusing upon what is not working. There is a power in focusing upon that which we want to create, rather than dwelling upon what we do not want.

David Wolfe, a leading expert in the Raw Food and nutrition movement, commented at a recent seminar: "Focus on your strengths and your weaknesses will take care of themselves."

Caroline Myss, a medical intuitive and leader in the personal transformation movement, tells an intriguing story that demonstrates the power of our thoughts. One time she was accidentally driven into the middle of a riot. Her young niece was with her and naturally the niece was frightened. Cars were being hit with baseball bats and overturned.

Myss turned to her niece and said, "*Whatever you do, don't think fear.*" A moment later, the men who were approaching their car with baseball bats suddenly turned and went a different direction. They placed their attention elsewhere. Coincidence? Maybe not. Perhaps a universal principle was at work.

You can only bring into your life that which is within your realm of belief. Creation cannot take place outside that realm; therefore, if you want to change your life you need to be willing to expand your belief system to incorporate new ways of looking at things. This is what I did on the day I chose a different course, the day I did not jump on the treadmill or blame my lover.

How do your beliefs impact your relationships?

If you believe you do not deserve to be treated well in a relationship or at work, you will not be treated well. If you believe you do deserve to be treated well, you will be treated well.

Is it magic? No. We are energetic beings and our thoughts and beliefs are energy as well. Our outer experiences are largely a reflection of our inner beliefs. There is a bit of a glitch, however, that we humans must overcome if we want to change our beliefs.

Sometimes our conscious beliefs are at odds with what we unconsciously believe. The very definition of unconscious is that it lies beneath the surface of our conscious mind. We are normally unaware of it. We cannot ordinarily access it.

The problem is the unconscious belief wins out over a conscious belief every time. The fact is that our unconscious beliefs are powerful and that we often hold on to self-defeating beliefs we don't even know we have.

If an unconscious belief is harming us, it would be valuable to know what the belief is so we can change it. We need a way to discover what our unconscious beliefs are before we can change them.

Since it is of the utmost importance to be able to gain access to these beliefs, the following chapter will introduce two techniques that can help you access and change any unconscious beliefs that may be holding you back. You can choose which beliefs you want to embrace, based on how they feel to you.

Personally, I have developed a standard I use to determine what I choose as a core belief. The question for me is whether the adoption of a belief will enable me to experience greater joy and happiness in my life. If so, I choose that belief. I believe that is a pretty good standard to follow.

How does all this relate to your body? If you believe that you are destined to be in a body that does not feel good to you, nothing can change. When you start to believe—and feel—otherwise, things will shift and wonderful experiences can begin to unfold in relation to your body.

Recognizing your ability to choose a beneficial belief gives you the opportunity to create a great life. You do not need to wait for someone to come along and present a great life to you (as if we are being served a great life as we would be served a meal).

We do experience life changes when we change our beliefs and therefore our way of viewing life. It is one of the more profound aspects of being alive that we have a degree of freedom and the power to alter the course of our lives.

Your life is largely your own creation. You may not control everything that happens, but you do control your response to what happens.

You get to create your unique life which is a reflection of your beliefs and choices. *The common denominator in all your life experiences is you. Choose beliefs that empower you.*

What Kind Of Relationship Do You Have With Your Body?

> **Just as you cannot thrive in a negative love relationship, your body cannot function well in the face of the onslaught of negativity you heap upon it. On the other hand, just as you thrive in a loving relationship, your body will thrive in a climate of love and appreciation.**

Think about your past romantic relationships. Have you ever been in a "bad" relationship? Chances are if you have been around awhile you know what it's like to be in a dysfunctional relationship. It does not feel good. Maybe you found yourself arguing a lot. Perhaps you said mean things to each other. You withheld from each other—affection or any positive emotion. Communication shut down.

You know, you've lost that lovin' feeling. The warm fuzzies have not been around for a long time. About this time you started talking with your girlfriends about all the things you did not like about your partner. It isn't pretty.

Now, think about your body and all the negativity you have been dumping on it, probably for years. The bottom line is this: *Good things do not come out of negative things. If you want your body to be good to you, you need to start being good to it.*

If you were in a relationship and you fed it negativity on a daily basis, would it thrive? If you then changed your approach completely and began to focus on the positive aspects of the relationship, would it change the nature of the relationship?

Well, you are in a relationship. The relationship is with your body. Your relationship with your body is the most intimate relationship you will ever have. We are interacting with our bodies on a moment-by-moment basis throughout our entire lives. *We need our bodies to live.*

Just as a relationship with a person might take awhile to come around when you stop the negativity and become more positive, so might your body need some time to come around.

Women have learned to think of their bodies in a peculiar way. This is always the case when we are out of balance. Distortions arise. On the one hand, as a woman you realize that your body captivates men. Your body is your gold, your bargaining chip. In that regard, you come to value your body as a way to "capture", and in some cases manipulate, men. Pardon my bluntness, but can it be denied that this sometimes is how it is?

In some religious contexts, although you might hear your body is your temple, there is also a teaching that "the flesh" is connected to carnal desire and that it is "bad." A real dilemma and something that completely messes up our heads because sexuality is core to being human.

The teaching that our natural body impulses are evil turns us against our very nature and ourselves. This is a terrible position to embrace and one that creates tremendous confusion and shame.

The application here is simply to recognize that we have warring factions inside when it comes to how we view our bodies. Our bodies are power, our bodies are seen as impure and debased.

In an odd way, we as women are taught to value our bodies and beauty because we realize they are the primary bargaining chip we bring to the table of life. It is our value as a woman.

Because of this, the pressure is great to possess a beautiful and "perfect" body. So much of our identity as women is placed on our body. Yet, ironically and understandably, it is often where we feel most insecure. We are never satisfied with our body. It is never quite good enough.

Look around and examine your own life and you will realize this is the truth. We are more neurotic about our bodies than any other aspect of ourselves. Why? Because it represents our ***desirability and value*** as a woman. How balanced is this?

You may value your body as a "calling card" to attract men, but it's more than that. Sure, it may be that it feel powerful to attract men (or women, if you love women). If *your entire sense of self-worth is limited to trying to have the best body ever, you are in for some serious disappointments.* Not to mention the possibility of a serious eating disorder. The best case scenario is you are going to age.

In order to let go of this neurosis about our bodies, we need to come into balance by coming to value and embrace all aspects of ourselves.

We are more than our bodies. We have a mind, emotions, and perhaps a spirit or soul. A well-rounded (read: happy & fulfilled) life involves developing your mental, emotional, and spiritual nature as well as coming to love your body.

One of the most empowering things you can do as a woman is balance your life by attending to these aspects of yourself, along with focusing upon your body.

Balance Your Life: Body-Mind-Emotions-Spirit

> **Women have a strange relationship with their bodies. We attribute our value as women to our bodies. Yet in overemphasizing their value relative to our status in life and obsessing over them, we don't actually love them.**
>
> **It is an odd paradox. Because our worth as women tends to be identified with our bodies, they matter to us greatly. Yet, exactly because our self-worth is so connected to our bodies, we become anxious and neurotic about them. We women are in a bind.**
>
> **Women's relationship with their bodies is in a state of imbalance—and this imbalance is a tremendous source of pain.**

What is the source of this imbalance? *We need to develop a more balanced relationship with our body and focus upon other aspects of ourselves as well. We need to incorporate all aspects of ourselves.*

Healing involves a willingness to come into balance. When we obsess about our bodies and ignore our other aspects, we've lost touch with our wholeness as human beings.

Although our body gives us our very life, and it is important to embrace it, the imbalance goes even deeper. We are required to do even more than come to value our body. We are called upon to ***value ourselves*** as human beings. This involves embracing all the aspects of our being and not over-focusing upon our bodies.

Think about it. Do you somehow view your body as being a separate entity from your self? Are you perceiving your body as separate from your mind, your emotions, your spirit?

The awareness that we are not separate parts, but rather one cohesive whole, has been the impetus for many healing modalities that incorporate "mind-body" healing practices. A recognition of this inseparable connectedness has now become mainstream. When we compartmentalize, divide, view life in a fragmented manner, we lose the wonderment of being alive.

Although it is beyond the scope of this book to evaluate the various philosophical and religious systems and their perspectives about the body, I would like to note that some systems of thought propose that the body is in some way inferior.

I would suggest that there is no such thing as a hierarchy when it comes to these functions. This bears repeating because to believe otherwise has created unnecessary pain and confusion.

No aspects of ourselves are "bad". *Any system that attempts to have you believe otherwise, that seeks to create a hierarchy making one aspect superior to the other, is distorted.*

Our body, mind, emotions, and spirit all contribute to and are integral aspects of who we are as humans. They cannot be separated and one is not "better" than any other. We cannot function as a whole without all these aspects. Any division we create is artificial.

All the aspects of you are valuable and necessary. In fact not one a*spect is more important than the other, all are intrinsic to our lives.* Without any of these aspects, we would not be human. Clearly though, without our body we would not have a life. How can we underestimate the significance of our bodies?

Even traditional medical practice acknowledges the importance of one's mental and emotional state in healing a so-called physical illness. We are encouraged to utilize visualization and keep a positive attitude, as it is widely regarded as invaluable to a healing process.

The holistic health movement recognizes the importance of integrating all the aspects of being human: physical, mental, emotional, and spiritual. We now know that emotions and experiences are stored in our muscles and tissues. Body work has evolved as a result of the mind and body working together, and an acknowledgment of the profound healing capabilities inherent in working with the body, mind, emotions, and spirit.

Think of the various aspects of yourself, recognize the value of your body (that allows you to be here and have every life experience you have ever had), and embrace the gifts of your mind, your emotions, and your spirit.

Your mind gives you the ability to think, to question, to expand, to make choices, to have options, to go beyond your conditioning. The mind becomes a problem only when it is not in balance.

Emotions are an intricate guidance system that allow you to know how you feel about any given experience. You have "gut" instincts that your emotions allow you to follow. Emotions allow you to feel, to love, to respond to life from the heart.

Your spiritual nature allows you to tap into the great mystery of life. Spirit is not about the specifics of what you believe. Rather, it is about the freedom of discovering your own inner truth and is a journey that is unique to you.

All aspects are valuable, not to be degraded in any way. It is when a particular aspect becomes imbalanced that distortions arise and we create problems for ourselves. Body-Mind-Emotions-Spirit. Each has a valuable function.

If we didn't need all these aspects, we would not have them.

If an aspect of our being was not of value, it would not exist. Doesn't it make more sense to embrace all our aspects and ***integrate*** *ourselves*?

What Story Are You Telling About Your Body?

Many of us are treating our bodies like they have no real value. Consider your possessions. You have possessions you absolutely love. No one could pry them away from you. You will *never* give them up. Those precious things are here to stay.

Now think about the things you have that you would gladly donate to the thrift store. *They have no value to you.*

How are you treating your body? Are you treating it like it is a prized possession or a thrift store item?

I would like you to think about something and try to be honest with yourself. Think about the many times you've repeated the same negative story about your body over and over. It can be to others or yourself.

Consider all the negative things you think and say about your body, including your shape and your assessment of your various body parts and features.

How many times have you put food in your mouth at the same time you say you shouldn't be eating it, or put yourself down as you talked about how fat or unattractive you are? If you are not overweight, think about all the other ways you have come up with to be unhappy with your body.

I have a few very important questions for you in relation to the negative stories you tell about your body:

- **How many times have you told these stories?**
- **Has your life improved as a result of telling these stories?**
- **Do you feel better as you tell these stories—or worse?**

Recognize that as you repeat the negative story you are reinforcing the current harmful paradigm. You are drinking the kool-aid and in the process betraying yourself.

Now consider this: *The stories you have told yourself about your body are false.* They are just stories. These stories are only true because you believe them to be.

Unfortunately, though, those stories are ruling you. Beliefs have a lot to do with what you create in your life. Your cells actually respond to your beliefs, as we've learned.

Do not feel bad as you realize how much you have participated in these negative stories. Remember you are not alone. The current paradigm, which has permeated our culture, thrives on these stories.

As mentioned previously, all you need to do is pay attention as you are going about your life. Whether in a café, a store, or at work, you are likely to hear women telling negative stories about their bodies on a regular basis.

Pay attention and see how long it takes before you hear such a story. More importantly, watch yourself and observe how often you tell the story.

A story is just a story. Yet, there is a significant risk involved. There is no inherent meaning or significance to a story except the meaning that we attribute to it. The emotion we experience and the meaning we attribute to the story is everything.

A story we tell ourselves long enough becomes a belief, and our beliefs largely determine the course of our lives. Therefore, be aware of the stories you are telling and the meaning you are attributing to them.

I am not that interested in your stories. Especially if they are hurting you. I find it more beneficial to guide you into creating more life-affirming stories. Your story is important, though, to the degree that it provides information that might be useful in helping you create a new story.

In order to do that, we do need to look at our current stories long enough to identify them so we know how to move forward. What story have you been creating about your body?

The new "stories" you can learn to tell are ones that help you to feel better about your body, yourself, and your life. They involve learning and practicing new ways of thinking and feeling about your body. The new stories have a lot to do with where you place your focus.

Rewrite The Story

If you want to have a different experience of your body, you need to rewrite your story.

As you begin to become aware of the stories you tell yourself about your body(and this is very useful for a variety of topics), you uncover the layers of beliefs that are embedded in your stories.

The power of uncovering these self-limiting beliefs is that you become more self-aware and can make other choices, creating a greater degree of empowerment and freedom. Empowerment is the ability to make life-affirming choices and to feel good about yourself.

If, as you think about your stories and beliefs about your body, you find that they are not serving you, it's a great opportunity to entertain the possibility that there is a more beneficial story you can embrace—one that will empower you to experience greater joy.

By becoming more aware you get to choose whether you want to continue acting out the limiting beliefs and suffer the consequences, or change the belief (the story) to one that can improve your life. You can then reap the benefits of your new beliefs, your new story.

Since your body is the most intimate relationship you will ever have, it benefits you greatly to make friends with it, to make peace with your body. Life is infinitely more enjoyable when you do. Making friends with your body allows you to begin to heal on many levels.

Loving your body is the foundation to loving yourself and the rest of your life. But, it is a foundation that's all too often non-existent and completely overlooked. This is a huge mistake. A foundation of loving your body is crucial to your overall well-being. You cannot love yourself without this foundation.

Identifying the current paradigm, utilizing the exercises in the Appendix, and uncovering your disempowering beliefs and changing them, will lead you into more beneficial stories naturally as you begin to recognize and embrace your body that gives you life and every wonderful experience you have ever had.

You come to know the real truth—that your body is your best friend. Create your story from that place and watch your life change.

CHAPTER THREE

Everything You Need To Know To Fall In Love

I prayed for the perfect thighs and my prayers were answered.
The answer was no.

—Leslie M. Murray

The Most Important Thing You Need To Know To FIL

Here is the most important piece of information I can give you about your body: *You would not be here without it. Well, that is a pretty obvious fact, is it not? Yet, perhaps you have never thought about that—and that's a big problem. One we are hopefully going to remedy!*

As obvious as this is, most people do not even consider it. Placing your focus upon this fact, and feeling it in the core of your being, is essential.

A change in how you think and feel about your body is what will enable you to experience a radical transformation in your life.

Reframing the way you think and feel about your body creates a paradigm shift as you come to recognize how magnificent your body truly is, and how much it wants to work well for you.

A very big part of reframing your perspective of your body is you getting it that *your body provides your very life.*

> **I cannot emphasize enough how important it is that you deeply understand and *feel* that you would not be here without your body. Your realization that your body gives you life itself has to take place in your core, not just intellectually.**
>
> **Thinking about it is not enough. It is just like giving a talk to drug addicts about how bad drugs are for their bodies—not effective. The habit is stronger than that. So it goes with our habit of negativity toward our bodies. We need to *feel* how good our bodies are to us, how valuable, how beloved, how central to life itself.**

Focusing in a new way is at the core of loving your body and involves perceiving your body in a completely new manner. It changes everything. *Where you place your focus says volumes about the quality of your life.*

Focus on the negatives about your body and you feel anxious and inadequate. Focus on the remarkable aspects of your body and you feel good, appreciative, and adequate.

As a result of changing your focus you can take a *huge* step in *freeing yourself from the anxiety and emotional pain* you feel about your body. You can begin to *relax* into your body in a new way.

Can you see how your negativity toward your body prevents you from truly feeling happy at your core? Your body is the most intimate aspect of you.

It's the only thing in your life that you carry with you wherever you go. Although I am stating the obvious, don't underestimate the power of it.

You are your body and your body is you. There is no separation, although you can become disconnected from your body and that's not a good place to live.

Your body attempts to work for you 24-7. Your body is a magnificent "machine," but evidence indicates it's a "machine" that responds to your thoughts. Since this is the case, it is of tremendous benefit to you to befriend your body!

We've already touched upon the obvious, but remarkable, fact that you would not be here without your body. Now, let's take it a step further.

Related to the fact that you would not be here without your body is another simple, yet incredibly profound insight: ***Every experience you have ever had is because you have a body. It is the very essence of being human.***

While this may sound—and is—basic, actually identifying with this has the power to change your entire relationship with your body in dramatic ways.

> **You will never appreciate your body until you realize it has provided both your life and everything you've ever experienced.**
>
> **If you take only two things from FIL let it be these:** *every life experience you have is because you have a body* **and** *you wouldn't be here without it.*

Everything else is secondary to these two realities. Embracing these simple facts can deeply change your life forever. It's rarely acknowledged and yet *without an appreciation of these two facts we can never truly love our bodies or ourselves.*

These two facts have been expressed in a variety of ways and in exercises that will help you to become keenly aware of how to incorporate them into your belief system and your life.

If you have felt bad about your body for a long time, you simply are not in touch with its magnificence. That is alright. In fact this is exactly why we are here, to create a new viewpoint.

You will begin to marvel at your body when you start to recognize that every wonderful thing you have ever experienced and enjoyed is because you are in this body.

Your body is the foundation of you. It is the vehicle that carries you through your life. *Without your body you would not exist!*

The most intimate relationship you will ever have is with your own body. It is the only thing that is with you every single moment of your life, from your first breath to your last. Yes, it bears repeating.

Where you go your body goes, where you are it is. Always! You are inseparable. Your body is not your enemy. Rather, your body is attempting to be your best friend. You are the only thing standing in the way.

Your body gives you life. The body is the foundation of existence in this physical, earth time-space reality. Your body works hard to keep you functioning every day.

By disliking our bodies we deny the vehicle that enables us to be here and experience every life event we have. Take this in.

As you begin to examine it, you will come to see the absurdity of being critical of your body. *It is truly "crazy making" to dislike our bodies.*

Cultivate a deep appreciation and reverence for your body—a truly amazing apparatus!

Learn to thank your body daily.

Inspired vs. Forced Action

Let's talk a little more about inspired versus forced action. My initial resistance to exercising or dieting in the moment my boyfriend told me he was no longer attracted to me due to my weight gain is now understandable.

It was not that there is anything wrong with exercise or eating well. Both can have tremendous value. But as with many things in life, the intention we hold when we perform an action makes all the difference in how much we benefit and our ability to continue long-term.

If we take forced action because we believe we must or out of fear or shame, it's more likely that we won't continue the action and make it a part of our daily lives. We don't enjoy it because we've *forced* ourselves to do it. We are doing it for the wrong reasons.

When we take action because we feel inspired, it is more likely that we will incorporate it into our daily lives with joy. We will ***want*** to perform that action. It's not forced because we feel embarrassed about our bodies. Rather it feels good because we love our body and want to do good things for it. Exercising and eating well can then become something that feels highly appealing.

The action is the same; but, the intention and emotion behind the action is different.

Falling in Love is about taking inspired, not forced action. Many of us have experienced the result of forced action. How often have you lost that 20 or 30 pounds? Is it lasting?

Why is it that the diet and exercise industries are multi-billion dollar operations; yet, at the same time, we have an extremely high rate of obesity in our culture? In combination with this are women in "perfect" bodies who are miserable and unhappy about them. We've had a real "number" done on us and we've bought it down to and at the expense of our hearts and souls.

While it is great to exercise, look good, and eat well, when balanced about it, eating well and exercise produce more lasting results when you're inspired. If not inspired, you'll tend to eventually fall back into old habits.

That's why a model for reframing how you view your body is a great adjunct to a healthy approach to eating and exercise. When you love your body you will naturally find yourself wanting to take care of it. This is a no-brainer.

Rather than forcing yourself into action, why not relax into well-being. Change doesn't require self-flagellation.

> **Exercising and dieting in a body one doesn't like is like giving your car an oil change when you need a new engine. It's not the best strategy ever. You are not addressing the real issue.**

Love your body first and everything else will fall into place. You may be amazed at what your body will do for you when you treat it with love and appreciation.

The My Life Will Be Better When Syndrome

How many times have you told yourself that your life will be better or that you will be happier when you have a "better" body?

The specifics of what you tell yourself regarding what would make for this "better" body are insignificant. We have an infinite number of ways to sabotage ourselves with the number of things we can come up with to criticize about our bodies.

The truth is that we already have and are everything we need to have and be in order to be happy in our bodies. *Being happy in our bodies— and our lives for that matter—is a state of mind.*

We believe we will be happy when we have the perfect body and this is an illusion. What we really want is to feel valued and loved. We long to love ourselves too, whether we know it or not.

These feelings are not the result of the perfect body. *Life is not necessarily better because we have a great body. Life is better when we love ourselves.*

Turn Your Attention Toward That Which You Seek

O ne key to loving your body more is to turn your attention toward that which you seek.

There is a reason that visualization is such a powerful tool. It's effective because the brain does not distinguish the difference between something "really" occurring and what we *imagine* to be real. This is a significant recognition and the application of it is useful in promoting change and in some cases even healing.

Because the brain does not distinguish between the actual and the imagined, it is extremely important to place your attention toward that which you seek and spend less time dwelling in thoughts that are negative or do not serve you.

It has been established that most of our thoughts are negative. If you examine where your mind goes throughout the day and listen to the conversation of others, it becomes clear that this is true.

Unless, that is, you *train yourself* to change the focus of your attention and thoughts. It is not hard to do this, but it does require a bit of effort and a little time.

Since most of us are in a "rut" regarding how we think about things—and specifically how we think about our bodies—rewiring our thought process and therefore our perspective is important. By being more mindful of the thoughts we "feed" ourselves, we can begin to experience an outlook that promotes greater well-being.

We start to become creators in our own lives, rather than being reactors. Reactors do what the word implies, react to all situations as if they have no control over what is happening in their lives. Therefore, nothing changes.

While it may be valuable to get in touch with and identify the negative self-talk you engage in with your body, as indicated we won't spend the majority of our time there.

Why? The answer is simple: You tend to get what you think about. For this reason it is important to *turn your attention toward that which you seek.* The opposite applies as well: *Turn your attention away from what you don't seek. What you focus upon tends to become your reality. Focus more on what you want to create and less upon what you don't want.*

We can almost become addicted to talking about and focusing on what is not working. This is so *habitual* that for many people it is hard to get them off that track.

You might know someone like this. No matter how much you may try to turn the conversation toward something positive they will return to the negative and talk about what's bad and wrong about their lives over and over. This is a toxic way to live.

Although the above example is extreme, we all tend to do this to some degree. Fortunately, we can train ourselves out of this habit as we learn to refocus in a different way. It takes a little practice, but is well worth it.

Creation begins with our thoughts. As we have talked about, thoughts become beliefs, and beliefs are reflected in the quality of life we're experiencing.

> **You may be thinking at this point it will be recommended that you turn your attention toward visualizing a perfect, beautiful body. Not so. Instead, *you are being encouraged to turn your attention toward falling in love with your body.***
>
> **There are already programs out there which use visualization to create the body and weight you desire. *Fall In Love* focuses differently and addresses the root cause of your discontent—which is how you feel about your body—and how to feel better.**

We have talked about identifying your self-talk because it can be a valuable tool to become more *aware* of what you are telling yourself, and because of this you have been encouraged to notice your thoughts and conversations about your body.

In turning your attention to thoughts and feelings about your body that help you feel good, you take the next step. You turn your attention toward that which you seek.

Love Is Not Only for the Thin

Many people who are not thin are under the mistaken assumption that they cannot have love (romantic love) unless they lose weight. Well, take a look around, girlfriends! Love is not reserved for the thin and being thin doesn't ensure you'll be loved.

People of all shapes and sizes experience love. If you believe that you cannot find love because of your body size, this is a story you are telling yourself that's simply not the truth.

One of my good friends is a great example. She does not fit the profile of the "perfect" body type in our culture. She is voluptuous, beautiful, engaging, and witty. She is definitely overweight by current standards.

The best part is that *she loves her body*! It is so interesting to observe people flocking to her. They are attracted like bees to the honey. She commands a room in moments.

Why? She radiates self-confidence. I am convinced that a large part of it is her love of her body. She feels sexy and most important *she knows her value.* My friend *knows* she's remarkable and she emanates this to others. She expects to be treated well and she is.

It has been said that self-confidence is the most powerful aphrodisiac. My friend is a wonder to behold and a great reminder to us all.

The most amazing piece of this story is how unusual it is to encounter a woman who truly loves her body, especially one who does not meet the "typical" standard of the ideal size.

Recently, a woman from Africa told me that her mother was distraught because her body size had decreased to a size 24. In many parts of Africa a larger body indicates wealth, as it means the person has plenty to eat. It's all about perspective.

Not only does the fantasy that only thin women are loved rob you of your now, it is simply untrue, which is why I call it a "bad" trick your mind plays on you. In the process, you rob yourself of your vitality and confidence as a woman.

Think about this. Do you realize that many women who are stunningly beautiful as defined by the cultural standard of beauty, and who have "perfect" bodies, feel inadequate and unhappy with their bodies? Many of these women feel unlovable, insecure in general, and lack self-esteem.

You may be one of those women. If so, you understand the pain involved. It is a lonely place to be. Beautiful women also face the wrath of other women who are jealous due to their own lack of self-esteem. It's sad what we perpetuate upon one another when we are not happy and empowered in our own lives.

Do you believe that love is reserved for only the most beautiful people in the most perfect bodies? Do you think they have the opportunity to have the "best" relationships or be loved the most? Take a look around. This is simply not true. Love is not reserved for any one body type or only the most beautiful.

Love is all around us.

> *One of the greatest mistakes we make is thinking of love as a commodity and one that is in short supply. On the contrary, love is not a thing, it is an experience that we generate inside. Love begins inside ourselves and radiates outward. As we love, we are loved.*

Having the "perfect" body or being the most beautiful is in no way an assurance that you will be loved more or experience greater happiness. The best assurance that you will be loved is in learning to love yourself. Your relationships will tend to reflect how you feel about yourself. If you value yourself others will value you. If you love and respect yourself, you will be loved and respected by others.

We tend to believe we will feel good when we have the perfect body. The truth is, though, it is not necessarily a "great" body you are seeking. You are seeking to feel valued, respected, and loved. The irony is that you first need to value and love yourself, not something we learned in school or at university.

Self-love is the magic formula.

The Story of Bacchus—A Life Lesson

I would like to share with you a story about my wonderful German Shepherd, Bacchus, that illustrates the power of belief and how important our beliefs are to what we experience.

Bacchus and I lived in Ojai, California, and we loved to go for walks out Creek Road. As the name implies, there was a lovely creek next to the road, and we loved to stop and play in it.

Bacchus loved water. If I turned on the shower in the house he would come rushing inside, run to the shower, and look up at the water with his tongue hanging out, his ears perked up, and tail wagging as if it were the most magnificent thing on the planet. He loved to play with hoses and would lunge for the water endlessly. One time he drank so much that he waddled home swishing. He looked a little peaked for awhile.

Well, the point is he *loved* water like there was no tomorrow, but the funny thing was *he didn't realize he could swim.* For weeks when we went out Creek Road I would test him by throwing branches into the water. He loved this game and would retrieve them happily.

Gradually, I would toss the branches out farther and farther into the creek trying to lure him to the place where the water was over his head. I would try to trick him into forgetting in the hope that he would accidentally swim and would then "get it" that he could indeed swim.

Bacchus did swim a few times accidentally, in those brief moments that he became so delighted in fetching sticks that he forgot himself and ended up over his head in the water. Amazingly, though, he never did "get it" that he could swim. And Bacchus was one smart dog.

I probably do not have to tell you the point of this story, but I will. My mind was fascinated as I watched him and coaxed him over weeks, to no avail.

I could not help but wonder: how many things could we do if we only knew we could, if we only believed in ourselves? If only we were willing to step out into the unknown with confidence and a sense of believing.

Never will I forget this experience and what it has taught me. Take the plunge. Be willing to take that next step. Move forward. Life is change. Change is growth. Growth brings joy. Trust the process. You can swim!

The Uniqueness of You

H ave you ever stopped to consider that there is no other you in the entire world? And there never will be! Reflect upon this the next time you are critical of yourself.

You are a unique being! Only you get to live your life, and your life path will largely reflect the views and beliefs that you embrace, consciously or unconsciously.

We become so preoccupied that we lose sight of some simple, yet profound, truths, such as the one above—you are unique! How awesome is that!

I remember years ago when I was experiencing a particularly painful period of my life. My father had just died after suffering greatly, and at the same time I experienced what seemed like a huge betrayal on the part of a trusted and loved person.

Although I consider myself a person with a very strong core, I felt truly "brought to my knees" spiritually and emotionally, one of those dark nights of the soul, as they say.

Sometimes late at night I would walk on the East End of Ojai with my wonderful German Shepherd Bacchus, on a moonlit night with a magnificent view of the mountains radiating the light of the moon. It was silent and beautiful.

On one of those evenings, middle of the night really, I remember thinking:

I may be in incredible pain and not know how I will move forward, but no one else gets to live my life. No one else gets to make choices for me. I get to live my life, I get to choose my responses.

It was a very powerful moment, as I realized that I had the opportunity to choose who to be. I get to respond to events in life. In fact, only I could choose my perspectives, beliefs, and responses to life.

This moment was one of the most freeing moments of my life. In the midst of tremendous pain, I realized the gift that was my life. The precious life that only I get to live.

This knowing—that you get to choose, that no one else gets to live for you—is powerful. The implication is that you are *free*.

Your uniqueness opens the possibility of freedom, you get to decide how to live. It is up to you to choose how you want to respond to circumstances, to each moment, to life.

The worst thing we can do is let others decide how our lives should look. Live your own life. It is your birthright.

You choose freedom by deciding you are going to embrace life and appreciate the gift that it is. Life can be bittersweet at moments. We experience losses. Yet, your life is yours and yours alone to live. Life is the best ever.

Think about this—you are walking around on the most magnificent planet in the solar system in your human form. Your uniquely human form is your "vehicle." You have been given this tremendous vehicle to accompany you through life, to provide a home for you, through this process we call life.

This is your body, remarkable almost beyond description. This body that performs literally thousands, millions, of "tasks" on a daily basis in order to keep you functioning. Be amazed!

And the next time you are walking on a beach, sailing on the ocean, watching a magnificent sunset, or gazing into the night sky and wondering whether there really are no boundaries, no ending to this universe, allow yourself to be touched by the elegance of this world, this universe, this body, and your unique life.

Take a look around. The beauty of this earth is astounding and you get to walk the face of it. What allows you to walk the earth, to experience everything you've ever experienced? Your body.

You are walking around in what might be *the* most sophisticated and evolved apparatus in existence. Wake up. Crawl into your body and cozy up to it. Your body is waiting for you. Your life is waiting for you. Claim it.

When you awaken to this reality, this knowing, this magnificence, a change occurs within you. You become more fully alive, more integrated, more in joy and wonderment. You begin to develop a natural appreciation for your body and your unique life.

This development is not forced in any way. Appreciation is a natural outgrowth of re-focusing and looking at things from a slightly different perspective. It is so very easy.

Belittling and criticizing your body, you lose touch with this very essence, the essence of the magnificence of your unique life and the life process that you are integral to and that is integral to you. You betray who you really are and the tremendous opportunity that has been afforded you.

Stop it! It no longer serves you. Choose differently. Claim your magnificence!

The recognition of the uniqueness of you, and the opportunity to be in your body and in your life, is a key aspect of loving your body. I wish for you to feel "on fire" in such a way that you will be excited about your life, not just your body.

Begin to love yourself, love your body.

The Turtle Story

There is a beautiful story in *The Tibetan Book of the Living and Dying* that presents a lovely analogy representing the preciousness of life, of being embodied. It's a story about the tremendous opportunity this physical life provides.

The story begins with an acknowledgment that inherent in many spiritual traditions is the belief that our lives as humans are unique and that our potential is beyond what we hardly begin to imagine.

The reader is encouraged to recognize that if we miss this unique opportunity to be in a physical body, it may be a long time before we have another opportunity of this nature:

Imagine a blind turtle, roaming the depths of the ocean the size of the universe. Up above floats a wooden ring, tossed to and fro on the waves. Every hundred years the turtle comes, once, to the surface. To be born a human being is said by the Buddhists to be more difficult than for that turtle to surface accidentally with its head poking through the wooden ring.

-Tibetan Book of the Living and Dying
by Sogyal Rinpoche (p.114)

I relate this story for the purpose of stimulating your awareness of how precious your life is. Regardless of specific spiritual beliefs, it is a beautiful perspective of life.

> *Do not sit around waiting for a great life to happen to you. That is an illusion. Create it. Your life is your gift and it is you who creates your life moment by moment.*

Loving Yourself

Chances are if you have explored personal growth you've heard a lot of talk about loving yourself. Loving yourself is the foundation upon which loving relationships are formed. Accepting and loving yourself, even with your human imperfections is central to having a good life.

The piece that is often overlooked is that if you do not love your body you can't love yourself. Think about it. Your body is an integral part of who you are. If you are critical of your body, you are critical of yourself. Yet, *ordinarily when one reads about self-love, loving the body is completely overlooked. This is a huge mistake.*

A couple years ago I was working on a book about relationships. The book on relationships evolved from another one of those personal "aha" moments I experienced as a result of a date.

I realized that by mid-life people still long for a love relationship, but they no longer believe it is possible. This puts them in a painful position. The initial part of the book was about self-love as the foundation for building loving relationships (and is part of my *The Fall In Love Process* series).

At the time I had already experienced the event that led to falling in love with my body, but had not made the connection to self-love and loving relationships (without self-love we cannot have the depth of loving relationships we are capable of).

Suddenly the realization occurred to me that for women particularly there is a step that needs to happen before we can love ourselves. That step is to accept, value and appreciate our bodies.

In other words, to truly love ourselves we must love our bodies. Not a small order of business considering how well trained we are to *not* love our bodies.

Recognizing the importance of addressing women's feelings about their bodies as the foundation to self-love, I decided to first write a book for women about their bodies and hence *The Body Program* was born.

> Loving our bodies is at the very core of self-love and love relationships. Self-love and loving relationships cannot be built without this foundation. A significant piece is missing and that missing piece will impact your overall relationship with yourself—and others. The missing piece is falling in love with your body.

The Value You Place On You

Perhaps the primary cause of pain in our human existence is a lack of love toward ourselves. Women especially have learned it is wrong and selfish to consider themselves, their own needs and wants.

As a woman, you are taught to value everyone else above yourself. Your training is to give until it hurts, without expecting anything in return.

Do you see how neurotic this is? If others are to be valued, doesn't it follow that you too deserve to be valued? And, believe me, if you do not value and love yourself no one else will. You set the tone for how you are treated.

You set the standard of your value. You set the bar. Others simply respond to your cues, albeit usually unconsciously. We train others how to treat us by an invisible agreement field that we have around us.

The agreement field of how we will be treated is reflected in how we treat ourselves, the value we place on ourselves, and our expectations in our relationships. You see, it's all up to you.

When we love ourselves others will naturally treat us better, for we expect to be treated well.

We probably all know someone who feels good about herself, and if you look at who they are with, you will notice that they tend to surround themselves with people who treat them well. Their partner, friends, and co-workers are good to them.

This is not an accident. Expectation is powerful. The value we place upon ourselves is not something we can fake. It's reflected in how we treat ourselves and in turn by those we surround ourselves with, especially in our close relationships.

We can build upon our sense of self-worth, though, and that is just what we are doing in *Fall In Love*. *Without examining our relationship with our bodies, there is no foundation for self-love.*

Each area of life affects the other areas. Virginia Satir, a prominent family therapist, used the analogy of a mobile to describe the impact family members have on one another. As she reached out and touched one part of the mobile all the other parts moved with it.

Satir indicated that this is what happens when one family member changes: It impacts the whole family system. This analogy applies to changes we make within ourselves as well. Each area of life we change impacts the other areas of our life.

As with the example of the mobile and families (touch one piece of the mobile and all the other pieces move with it), changing one aspect of your life will impact other areas of your life.

Imagine how your relationship with others and your overall outlook and attitude toward life could change if you stopped disliking yourself (your body) and began to appreciate, maybe even adore, your body.

One change is that you may find yourself not being so dependent upon what others think of you—your appearance or otherwise. It is wonderful to have nurturing relationships, and we thrive in them. It is also a great feeling to know that your sense of self-worth is not totally dependent upon what others think.

If we remain alienated from our bodies we cannot truly connect in a manner that leads to a fulfilling and remarkable life. This is a strong statement, but look around and ponder this.

You are the most important person in your life. Your life matters. You need to become the most important person in your own world. If you do not consider yourself to matter, you don't have a whole self to offer others and are limiting your own joy and the contribution you could be making.

Likewise, if you are not loving your body you are fragmenting yourself and therefore are not fully available to yourself or others.

Valuing and loving yourself and your body is a perspective. It's a matter of generating a feeling inside yourself. It is for this reason that one often hears "if you want to experience love, emanate love."

Self worth is not generated from the outside in, but rather from the inside out. Your outer life is a reflection of your inner world.

Transformation At Your Fingertips

Transformation is not only possible, it is at your fingertips. Every moment holds a possibility for change, a new viewpoint, a different perspective. You have so much choice that it's astounding.

Abraham-Hicks stated:

> *What provides more freedom than a world in which we are free to choose our own thoughts? There can be no greater freedom than the freedom to choose our thoughts, our perceptions.*

It is fascinating to recognize that we have a tremendous capacity for transformation that can be applied not only to our relationship with our bodies, but also in other relationships and to life in general.

You hold all the power. It's truly remarkable when you recognize this truth. The power you hold is the power of self-empowerment, the ability to choose, to create your life or at least guide the course of it, with your responses. The ability to respond to a situation out of choice, rather than simply reaction, is key to a mature emotional life.

We give away our power by holding beliefs and perspectives that do not benefit ourselves or others around us. Unfortunately, we then blame outside forces (such as the beauty industry, men, our families) and see ourselves as the victim or martyr, not recognizing that we are creating the problems.

Blaming others is a fantasy that can create tremendous misery and confusion when we're not aware it is self-created. Fortunately, we can take our power back by recognizing the thoughts and emotions that are harming us and changing them.

Empowerment largely relates to our ability to guide our own destiny. We are not pawns in this life, but rather active participants. If you fail to recognize this, though, it will feel like life is living you rather than you living life.

This is not meant to imply that difficult things don't occur in life. They do. This constitutes the ebb and flow of life. Loss is part of life. Yet, regardless of your life experiences, you get to interpret and formulate the meaning you give those experiences. The way you do this reveals a great deal about the quality of life you are likely to be living.

The great news is you can choose to change the meaning and doing so can alter the course of things dramatically. You do this by changing your point of focus and changing your beliefs. This is transformation.

Although it may be difficult at first to come to terms with the thought that you largely create your life experiences through your beliefs, it can actually be a freeing perspective to embrace. It gives you the opportunity to feel more empowered and to create something more wonderful in your life.

I bring this to your attention because I want you to begin to realize that you can do this! You can change your perspective of your body in such a way that it will free you to experience greater joy and feel a sense of incredible appreciation for your body. In so doing, how you feel about yourself will change—and I believe it is a change you will love!

There is no need for you to be in a body that you feel ashamed or embarrassed about. While I cannot promise that those feelings will never arise—we have been incredibly conditioned for many years—I can promise that if you embrace some of the concepts we are addressing here you will have the tools to create lasting change in your life. If or when you get off track you can utilize these tools to get back on track.

The exercises are transformational. You can practice them wherever you are. It does not even require a pen and paper or a computer. Although I recommend you write them out initially, eventually these concepts will become hard-wired in your brain, in the manner that your negative concepts about your body are currently hard-wired. You are changing the software.

Once this happens, when you start "running" the negative tapes (stories) in your mind, your brain will have had enough experience of perceiving in another way—more embracing, supportive, and loving—that you will quickly notice.

You will change your self-talk to that which is more life-affirming and brings you greater happiness, you will remember who you are. It simply takes some practice.

Transformation is at your fingertips.

CHAPTER FOUR

Fall In Love With Your Life

True freedom and the end of suffering is living in such a way as if you had completely chosen whatever you feel or experience at this moment.

—Eckhart Tolle

The following segments provide excellent information, perspectives, and practices to help you improve how you feel and to create a more aware and happy life.

The more "awake" you become, the more likely you are to feel good about your body, yourself, your relationships with others, and being alive.

Awakening is simply becoming more conscious and aware. The information in this chapter is meant to help you awaken.

The Fall In Love Process is about feeling good in all areas of your life. The information that follows can help you feel better from the inside out.

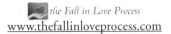

Living in the Now

A good life is comprised of a series of good moments. Yet we chase a good life by looking toward the future and hoping that somehow amazing things are going to drop into our laps. By living in the future we miss the juicy NOW moments that make for a good life.

It's like a trick the mind plays on us to constantly live in—or dwell in—the past or future rather than be present in the moment. *The problem is the past cannot be changed and is forever gone. The future is an illusion, a fantasy that never arrives.* The future is a self-created myth. We can't know what the future will bring.

Now is what we have. Yet, if we are not fully present, we miss out on our life. **Now is the place where life resides.**

Realizing that a good life is made up of a series of good moments is one of the most profound things you could ever grasp.

I recall a particular experience I had that caused me to realize I wasn't being present in the moment. I was at an outdoor concert where there was a large group of people. As I have moved a few times, my friends are scattered throughout the country and world. I have always had time periods in which I do things by myself and I am usually quite comfortable with it.

At this concert, though, I found myself fantasizing about how much more enjoyable it would be if I had a friend or partner there with me at that moment. If the truth be told, I was feeling a little sorry for myself.

It was interesting for me to observe my own thought process and become aware of what I was doing. My focus on wishing for something different was preventing me from being fully present in the experience.

Once I realized that I was focusing on how I imagined I would have liked it to be—and in doing this was missing the opportunity to enjoy the moment as it was—my perspective changed. I immediately made a choice to be in the moment exactly as it was and as if by magic it shifted my experience. I began enjoying the people around me and the experience of the concert. I had a great time.

Although this is one small example, the practice of being present and available to the moment has tremendous implications for the quality of your life. Being present in the moment means that wherever you are, whatever you are doing, and whomever you're with, you are giving your attention to it. You are not in a fantasy about the past, the future, or what you wish you were doing.

If you can apply being fully present in the moment to your life, your happiness quotient is likely to rise exponentially.

Let's take a moment to translate this as it relates to thoughts about your body. Many of us fantasize a future when our bodies are the size we want or look the way we want, and think we will then become happy. Promoting this fantasy prevents you from experiencing joy *now*. You are always waiting for a future moment—and that moment may never arrive.

It's a trick the mind plays upon you. For many people this fantasy goes on for years and years. **While engaging in this fantasy, you're missing out on your life!**

Not only does this fantasy rob you of now, it is simply untrue, which is why I call it a "bad" trick your mind plays on you. Even if you achieved the so-called "perfect" body, this is no guarantee of happiness. Thin women with perfect bodies are not all having the happiest of lives and many larger women are living happy lives.

Feeling good is a state of mind and heart. Come into the present. Life is in the now.

The Language of Woundology: Are You Speaking It?

Caroline Myss made a fascinating discovery about a common way that people relate. She calls it speaking the language of "woundology." The purpose of including it here is to enable you to identify whether you are speaking this language and change to something more empowering if you are.

In her profound book and audio program called *Why People Don't Heal*, Myss describes this language in depth. She observed that most people relate with one another by talking about their wounds, things they are unhappy about, and traumas they have experienced. Woundology often involves *blaming others* for our problems as well.

In fact, her contention is that we not only relate on this level, but **we bond with others around our traumas.** *Bonding over our wounds can be almost as powerful as a drug.* Bonding around our unhappiness and traumas creates a feeling of comfort and closeness with others

We don't have to look far to discover that indeed many conversations focus on negative and painful topics. Chances are that you have participated in many of these types of conversations. I know I have.

The point is not that it isn't good to give and receive support or sometimes need help from others. Rather, it is realizing that when we become largely **identified** with our hurts and wounds, it is disempowering and negatively impacts the quality of our relationships and our life.

In essence, this habit can keep us frozen in a place in which personal growth is not possible. We become stuck and victims of life, rather than co-creators.

Myss uses the analogy of therapy or gaining support from our friends as taking a boat across a river. Getting stuck in speaking the language of woundology is akin to not making it across the river. It keeps us in a victim/martyr role.

As women, we are frequently indoctrinated to take on the victim/martyr role, feeling that others are to blame for the things we experience in life. We learn to devalue what's important to us and then blame others when we take care of everyone but ourselves.

There is nothing less attractive than playing the victim/martyr card. It does not make for an oh so happy life. Yet, it is a role many of us learned well and for good reason.

You may have "legitimate" arguments for feeling like a victim. Still, the question becomes "how does it make you feel to be a victim or martyr?" If it doesn't feel good, it is time to do something different.

Speaking the language of woundology doesn't take you where you want to go if what you want is a better feeling life.

The truth is you and only you have the power to change your life, but there is a catch. *In order to have the power you need to give up playing the victim.*

The first step toward change is identifying whether you speak the language of woundology and owning that it is not working for you. The language of woundology keeps you in a life that's less than good.

You can choose to change your perspective—and in the process change the quality of your life. Naturally though, you need tools to engage in a change process. You cannot get across the river without the oars.

You need to re-train yourself into a more empowered way of viewing your body. Become aware of the language you are speaking, in relation to your body and your life.

Blaming (the language of woundology) will get you nowhere, except feeling hopeless and disempowered.

Real power is not about controlling others, it's about having the capacity and will to direct the course of your own life. *In order to heal you must stop blaming anyone or anything and take 100% ownership over how you feel and own your ability to change your life.*

If you blame something or someone outside yourself, you are powerless. You cannot make that person or society change. The only thing you can change is you. That's very cool because *it places all the power in the one place where you can have an impact—within yourself.* And that is all you need. It is the jackpot.

It does not really matter how we got here. What matters is you (we collectively) are here. *The real question is: What are you going to do about it?*

I have got to give it to you straight because I care too much to water it down. My desire is to awaken you out of the stupor, to interrupt the status quo that we have all bought into that keeps women disempowered. Disengage the autopilot. *You deserve more!*

Are you ready to take your power back? Stop speaking the language of woundology.

> **With each thought, each emotion, each conversation about our bodies, we are either creating further disillusionment and pain, or greater happiness, satisfaction and joy. Let us stack the odds more in favor of joy by being aware of our thoughts, emotions, and conversations and choosing a bit more wisely.**

Are You In Charge Of Your Life?

I n psychology there is a concept called **locus of control**. There are two styles of locus of control; people fall into one of two categories. The two styles are called external and internal locus of control, and they portray a person's worldview.

People who adhere to the external model believe that they don't have control over their lives, that events just happen to them.

Individuals who adhere to the internal locus of control believe they do have control over what happens in their lives, that they can have some degree of impact on their life circumstances.

Which group do you believe lives a more satisfying life?

Naturally, it is the group who believes they have some degree of power over their lives. I believe that to a large degree we can shift our locus of control by shifting our focus and beliefs.

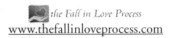

The Trances We Live In

O ur mental and emotional states may be likened to trances. We often think that hypnosis and going into trance is some sort of magic tool or unusual occurrence. Stephen Wolinsky, PhD., points out in his excellent book *Trances People Live*, that one way of viewing trance is as a state that results in a narrowing of attention in a way that limits our options.

Here are some examples of states: Joy is a state. Anxiety is a state. Depression is a state. Obsessiveness is a state. Playfulness is a state. Rage is a state. Appreciation is a state. *Which states do you prefer and are you experiencing them as often as you would like?*

A trance state by its nature decreases our attention on other things. We become super focused a particular state and other things fall into the background. We all have areas in which we tend to become "fixated." During those times, we are in a sort of trance (the words trance and state can be used interchangeably).

Our thoughts and feelings about ourselves or a particular situation or relationship become "fixed," and we become unable to maneuver into more expansive ways of viewing the situation.

Wolinsky provides a great analogy for these states and explains them in this way:

The mind is like a library. Within this library are numerous sections. For example, we have a body section, a job section, a relationship section. At any time we can retrieve a particular section by shining a flashlight (that is, our awareness) on it.

Wolinsky makes the point that all sections are there at all times, but we can only take a look at a certain section if we place our mental focus upon it.

We enter these states or library sections, usually unaware, by allowing our emotions and thoughts to take on a life of their own. They become automatic, and in doing so we lose our sense of choice.

At these times, we do not recognize opportunities to maneuver into different viewpoints. We often form these states as a way to deal with trauma and shield ourselves, particularly in childhood. While going into these "trances" initially assists us in coping with trauma, it later becomes a detriment due to its habitual nature.

This becomes obvious if one examines the fact that these "states" narrow our range of possibility and choice. These areas are often issues or situations that "trigger" us, push our buttons.

Think about an area of your life in which you tend to become "triggered" and react without thinking or consciously deciding. Consider something that you tend to ruminate and perhaps even obsess upon—maybe your body!

These are areas where we can be pretty certain we are going into "trance", i.e., narrowing our attention and focus to the point where we lose the bigger picture. We lose the ability to perceive a more inclusive way of seeing something. We really believe that what we are telling ourselves is the truth when in actuality we're limiting ourselves.

Another way of becoming aware of the key issues—and perhaps a good way to get in touch with specific examples—is by noticing your self-talk, the things you say to yourself. Becoming aware of the negative self-talk or chatter in your mind helps you to identify your "trance" material.

Sometimes our self-talk is directly related to things we were told about ourselves as children. We then internalize these messages (whether spoken or inferred) and begin to tell this to ourselves. It becomes our story.

If the "story" is a negative one, it becomes self-perpetuating and we are unable to step outside of this story to entertain a different perspective or approach without assistance. If we're unable to expand our story, we become trapped in negative self-defeating beliefs (stories). Creating a new story is one way of describing stepping out of the trance into a more beneficial emotion and viewpoint.

Our limiting beliefs are another "clue" relative to trance states. Some examples of a negative "trance" state might be the belief that we are never going to amount to anything, that we or others are untrustworthy, that we cannot have a decent relationship, are basically flawed, aren't smart, are too fat, and no one will ever be attracted to us.

You get the picture. The disempowering "stories" (or trances states) we can tell ourselves are endless and the result is a sense of dysfunctional relationship patterns, disappointment, and emotional pain.

Wolinsky notes that the real work in therapy is noticing when we are in a particular trance (which limits our ability to respond) and learning to shift our trances or "states" to more expansive and encompassing states, allowing for greater choice. Becoming aware of limiting beliefs and changing them is one way to do this. Accessing unconscious beliefs and shifting them is particularly beneficial, especially considering the power they often hold over us.

In order to love your body, it is important to begin to recognize the trances you are experiencing relative to how you think and feel about your body (think the current body paradigm beliefs, the status quo, drinking the kool-aid). Clues as to how you feel about your body can be gleaned by becoming aware of your thoughts about it—what you tell yourself about it—as well as the feelings you have about it. How you talk with others about your body also provides valuable clues.

A remedy for negative beliefs about your body is to broaden and expand your focus, so that you might embrace more life-affirming perspectives and allow for a greater experience of well-being. Specifically, you need to create new "stories" to counteract the negative stories you have been telling yourself about your body.

The Fall In Love Program teaches you how to cultivate a specific state within yourself in reference to your body. The exercises are the best tool you can use. You are doing them, right?

One effective tool for dealing with states that we want to change is to use the witnessing technique, which is discussed in the next section.

Although I have briefly described a couple key concepts in Wolinsky's work (I would highly recommend his book, as we have just touched the surface), many others in the personal growth arena have focused on similar concepts. We have a tremendous amount of information and tools available for our personal growth and to change to more empowered and enjoyable states.

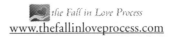

Witnessing: A Process For Self Awareness

Our minds constantly create thoughts. If you have ever practiced meditation, you know that one of the first things you notice—and are encouraged to pay attention to—is the steady stream of thoughts that go through your mind.

In Eastern religions and philosophies there is a practice of mindfulness training called witnessing. Witnessing involves the developing the habit of becoming a conscious observer of your own thoughts and emotions.

As you become more aware of your thoughts and feelings, you begin to realize that you are more than these thoughts and emotions. They move through you but they are not you. There is a you behind your thoughts and emotions. You are more. As you notice this, your identification with your thoughts and emotions tends to decrease.

As a conscious observer we tend to be more detached from our thoughts and emotions than when we're not noticing them, but rather just "in" them. The act of mindfulness and self-awareness in itself creates an opportunity to view things from a slightly different perspective.

Mindfulness through witnessing, or being the observer, affords you the opportunity to make different choices. It is like stepping back and watching yourself from a distance. This slight distance allows a bit of detachment that can help you see things differently, becoming less identified with your thoughts and feelings. This can help you take a more balanced approach toward them.

Becoming more mindful, more aware of your thoughts and feelings, helps you create a better life. Witnessing or mindfulness is a technique to assist you to see the seer behind the seeing, the thinker behind the thought. *You realize you are more than your thoughts and emotions.* They are not the totality of who you are.

Meditation is a tool you can use to observe and become aware of thoughts and emotions. Simply becoming more aware of your thoughts and feelings throughout your day and knowing you are more than this, is another practice you may utilize.

Witnessing your own process through mindfulness practice allows you to experience your life in a more aware manner.

How To Make Affirmations More Effective

Affirmations in themselves lack the power to create significant change unless you join the thought with a strong emotion. A thought without emotion has little impact; however, a thought coupled with emotion has a tremendous impact.

We respond to how we feel about something more powerfully than what we think about it. This is why affirmations are not effective if we haven't generated a feeling that matches the words we are saying. This is the case whether the emotion is positive or negative.

For this reason, as you affirm something it's important to create a positive emotion by envisioning and actually feeling how it will be when you experience what you're affirming. Generate the feeling of what you want and imagine how you will feel when it occurs. In fact, *imagine it as if it is happening now.* Visualization is processed in the brain in the same manner as an actual event, as we've already noted.

The combination of thought coupled with strong emotion significantly increases the benefit of affirmations. A great resource for learning this technique and other beneficial ways to experience what you want in life is the Abraham-Hicks material by Esther Hicks. See the Resource Section of this book for this information.

We do not need to set goals in order to change our lives. Rather, what is needed is a change of perspective. It really is this simple, although this runs contrary to a prevailing notion that we need to set goals and then work long and hard toward meeting those goals.

Changing a belief changes our experience. As our beliefs shift relative to our bodies, we create new life-affirming experiences. *Fall In Love* isn't about hard work, but rather embracing and relaxing into greater well-being. Spend a few moments a day envisioning the feeling of how you want to feel in your body.

It feels good to feel better about our bodies and envisioning and affirming how we want to feel is a great tool. As we begin to feel better a momentum is built that leads to a greater sense of well-being. These positive feelings build upon themselves as we create more and more positive experiences.

> **Visualize how you want to feel. Visualization is a powerful tool. Notice I did not say envision how you want your body to look. Rather, it's about how you want to *feel* in your body. If you focus only upon how you want your body to be you're missing the boat completely. You have not built the foundation that is at the core of stepping out of the current body paradigm that keeps you feeling anxious and insecure about your body.**

Relative to loving your body, stay with your vision until you feel the good feelings about your body in the core of your being. A great way to do this is to write the exercises (which put you in a good feeling place about your body) and close your eyes, allowing these feelings to wash over you.

At the end of the exercises you're introduced to a technique called *anchoring* which helps you incorporate these feelings into your body in a way that you can re-access them at any time.

The reason so many programs about the body fail is they are going at it from the wrong direction. Putting the cart before the horse so to speak. The foundation of self-love is missing.

You need to fall in love with your body now rather than pretending to yourself that you'll love your body when it becomes perfect.

That elusive when . . . Step out of the fantasy and claim the life you were meant to have now.

the Fall in Love Process
www.thefallinloveprocess.com
100

The Power of Appreciation

Gratitude is a word that is likely to make you yawn when you read it. There was a time when I thought it was boring too. That was before I started practicing appreciation.

Years ago I began a daily practice of beginning my day by writing all the things I felt appreciative of in my life. It could be anything from having a place to live, good food to eat, having work I loved, to the beauty of the tree that I was seeing out the window.

The content of appreciation is not important, but gratitude is perhaps one of the most significant change processes you could practice.

I was stunned at the power of my gratitude practice. My perspective changed dramatically. I began focusing upon more and more aspects of great things to appreciate. How I felt changed. My life was transformed by my daily gratitude practice—and that is not an exaggeration. After a time, I automatically found more and more throughout my day to appreciate and enjoy.

As my appreciation for life increased dramatically, I began experiencing numerous serendipitous encounters. I'd think about something I wanted and the next thing I knew it was at my fingertips effortlessly. If there was someone I needed to see for some reason, they would show up.

You may recall that Dr. Lipton stated the best thing we can give our cells is love. A gratitude practice will have you loving life. I cannot overemphasize how beneficial this practice can be. It's a great antidote for negative thinking.

After awhile, you naturally begin to focus on what feels good and what is working. You have re-trained your mind and your life will reflect this. Try it and see for yourself. It is one of the best things you can do for your well-being.

What Promotes Healing?

After decades of working in the mental health arena, I am convinced that profound change and healing does not usually occur by simply talking about our problems. While it may be beneficial to become more aware of our patterns, awareness alone often does not promote change and healing. It can be a great first step but more is required.

The most important question about therapy in my mind has been "What promotes healing?" *If something does not promote healing, then clearly it's not a beneficial path to follow.*

My experience, both professionally and personally, has led me to believe that healing occurs through modalities that utilize both mind and body together. For some individuals a spiritual component is an aspect of healing as well.

Mind-body work does not require a mental understanding for healing to occur. That is why figuring things out doesn't necessarily help you feel better.

Unconscious beliefs have a powerful influence upon us, yet we usually are not aware of them. In fact, that is the very definition of unconscious, it means something that is not in our awareness.

Conscious thoughts and beliefs are those we have access to in our everyday awareness. That is why they're called "conscious." The nature of unconscious beliefs is that we are unaware of their presence.

It has been said that if you want to be aware of your unconscious beliefs, take a look at your life. Examine the different areas of your life and assess what you are experiencing in each important area: relationships, money, work, body, self-esteem, and any other area that is meaningful to you.

In order to change your unconscious beliefs that may be harming you, you need to know what they are. In the next chapter you'll be introduced to two different techniques to access your negative unconscious beliefs and change them to more self-affirming ones.

CHAPTER FIVE

Mind-Body Healing Techniques: Access & Change Your Unconscious Beliefs

The level of thinking that created the problem is not the level of thinking that will resolve the problem.

—Albert Einstein

These days there are so many tools available for healing that there is no reason to live in a place of pain and disempowerment.

We are living in a remarkable time and have numerous mind-body tools available for healing. The following two techniques are reviewed due to their powerful ability to help you heal any area of your life where you are blocked and not living your full potential. I have utilized both these techniques in my own life and have found them to be incredibly beneficial.

The first tool is called *Emotional Freedom Technique (EFT)*, commonly called "Tapping". The healing power of this simple technique and its various applications is remarkable.

Emotional Freedom Technique (EFT) In A Nutshell

EFT involves tapping lightly on certain meridian points (energy points) on the body. As you tap you construct simple sentences that describe the "problem" you wish to address and use them as you "tap" on these energy points.

You can tap on any issue that negatively impacts your life—health, money, pain, relationships, self-love, body issues, anxiety, and phobias. Tapping is easy and you can learn the basics quickly. Most importantly, *it bypasses the conscious mind.*

EFT sometimes **clears phobias** *within minutes*, although it may take more time. It's been used for *Post Traumatic Stress Disorders* effectively, often with veterans returning from combat. EFT may help *reduce physical pain* and is used to treat *anxiety.*

You can use EFT to **clear emotional issues** that you may have been dealing with for a long time. You can tap your way to improved *self-esteem, improved relationships,* and *loving your body and yourself.*

Tapping may help you clear a lot of the negative things you have believed about your body all these years by adopting the current body paradigm.

I know, *it sounds really weird.* Yet, think about the benefits of acupuncture and acupressure. Acupuncture works with the meridian points as well and you know it is effective when you see someone wide awake chatting through a heart surgery with just a few needles in their ear!

Significantly, traumatic memories and limiting beliefs are stored in our bodies. We are comprised of energy and *the flow of energy through your body can become trapped.* EFT opens your energy channels and releases blocked energy and emotions. Releasing the energy benefits you both physically and emotionally.

The greatest thing about EFT is that after a little practice, you can do it yourself. That means even if you don't have a lot of money to spend on therapy, you can readily learn it and use it on your own. This is tremendously empowering as it places your healing in your own hands. EFT offers people the ability to experience healing even though they may not have financial resources.

EFT is a potentially life-altering tool. Tapping is a simple, yet effective way to dramatically improve the quality of your life.

As noted, it is *something you can learn easily and apply on your own.* I love that about EFT. You can do it anytime and anywhere *you* choose. Translate this as a tool that's always at your disposal. You don't have to wait until you have an appointment with a therapist. A lot of money is not a prerequisite.

EFT bypasses the conscious mind and is a mind-body tool. *Mind-body modalities utilize the wisdom of your body and recognize the connection between body and mind.* Bypassing the conscious mind is a significant aspect in healing.

Your well-being depends upon you having empowering information and techniques that you can utilize on your own.

I have been amazed at the power of this simple tool. I've experienced that I can almost immediately tap into emotions I did not even know were there. It simply feels like a great release of energy. And that is exactly what it is.

That's why it's called Emotional *Freedom* Technique. You release into a sense of greater well-being. You feel lighter in your being as you open up energy that has been blocked in your body.

Specifics of the Technique

A wealth of information is available on the Internet that explains how tapping is done. Rather than repeat the information here, I am going to steer you toward a few great websites on EFT that I hope you will enjoy. Several sites are available that describe EFT in depth, including videos to show you the technique, as well as explaining the various uses for EFT. You can also check out videos on YouTube.

Initially it is best to find a practitioner near you and *go to a few group or individual sessions to learn first-hand how tapping is done.* You can then begin using it independently.

Here are a few EFT websites:

> http://www.eftuniverse.com
> http://tappingcentral.com
> http://www.thetappingsolution.com

PSYCH-K: Access & Change Your Unconscious Beliefs

A great way to access unconscious beliefs is through a process called PSYCH-K.

I first was introduced to PSYCH-K when I read leading edge cell biologist Bruce Lipton's book: *The Biology Of Belief.* Lipton points out, as previously mentioned, that we are *not* ruled by our DNA, but rather react to our *perceptions* of our environment. *Our cells respond to our beliefs.*

In other words, we respond to our *beliefs* about what we are experiencing and how we perceive what is taking place around us. In this process our cells are impacted for better or worse. Even traditional medicine now recognizes that attitude and our thoughts significantly impacts whether we heal from an illness.

Lipton describes a dilemma: although he discovered the profound impact our beliefs have upon our biology, he did not know how to change a harmful belief. A serendipitous encounter provided the answer that changed his own life. He heard a lecture by the founder of Psych-K, Robert M. Williams.

PSYCH-K is a method to access the unconscious mind in order to create profound change *easily* and often *rapidly*. Because our unconscious beliefs can have a negative impact on our lives, it is essential to have a technique to access them and replace them with more life-affirming beliefs.

As I have mentioned, as a psychologist, I've always wondered *what actually promotes change and healing.* We now know that *talking about problems with a therapist may help you become more aware, yet awareness does not necessarily bring change.*

the Fall in Love Process
www.thefallinloveprocess.com
108

Since PSYCH-K allows you to access your unconscious beliefs, let's look at a couple areas of life where your unconscious beliefs may be harming you. Let's examine your beliefs relative to relationships and money.

Relationships are an area where people often struggle to overcome unconscious beliefs. You may consciously *think* you deserve a loving romantic partnership, yet you may tend to become involved in relationships in which you're not treated well and feel disregarded, not seen or valued. *This is a cue that unconsciously you probably do not actually believe you deserve a loving partnership.*

Perhaps while growing up you never saw an example of a loving relationship and emotional pain may be "tied in" with your perception of a romantic relationship.

In extreme, we often witness people who grew up in abusive households experiencing abuse in their adult relationships. A pattern has been set into place that we tend to repeat. In this case the pattern is that love has come to be coupled with abuse and therefore love = abuse. Rarely is this a conscious belief and yet the impact can be devastating.

Finances is another area where many people struggle.

Ask yourself this question: *Do you believe you are worthy of having enough money to be comfortable financially?*

Now, consider your actual current financial situation. *Do you have enough money that you are comfortable financially? If you think you're worthy of having enough money and yet don't, that means your conscious belief about money most likely does not match your unconscious belief.*

You may *think* you deserve to have money, yet your life may be filled with lack of money. *Your lack of money indicates that you most likely have an unconscious belief that is in conflict with your desire for money.*

Maybe growing up your parents said that people with money are selfish, cold, or uncaring. Or, perhaps in your family the message was given that money is very hard to come by and that you always need to struggle just to make ends meet. It may be that deep down you are afraid people will not like you if you have money or you may believe unconsciously that you don't deserve to be provided for.

Money represents value. Outwardly you may think you should have money and cannot figure out why you don't. The reason often is that your desire for money is overshadowed by your unconscious beliefs about it. This can be true relative to any area of your life.

The point is, regardless of the source or specific issue, our unconscious beliefs are more powerful than our conscious beliefs. *If you want to see what you really believe, take a look at your life.* Examine your life for clues as to what you really believe.

Your unconscious beliefs will take the driver's seat and "run" your life every time!

For example, In the money scenario, it is your unconscious belief you are not worthy of having money that may be creating the scarcity of money in your life.

Look at your money situation, your romantic and family relationships, friendships, work, and your body to discover what you actually believe about these areas of your life. Accessing your self-defeating unconscious beliefs allows you to begin the process of healing your life and feeling better in all the areas mentioned.

If you want to know what your beliefs are take a look at your life.

Your *conscious mind* stores all the thoughts and beliefs you *think* you hold about your life. *You're aware of these thoughts* (hence the term conscious).

Your *unconscious mind,* on the other hand, holds all the beliefs that run the show. *In other words, your unconscious mind is basically controlling your life!* These beliefs are hidden underneath the surface. You are not aware of them. They are like the software of a computer and have infinitely more power over your life than your conscious mind. *They simply keep running the same "tapes" over and over unless something intervenes.*

You know what I'm talking about. *The "stuff" that you keep doing or experiencing over and over and wonder "What the hell's going on here? I know better!"* At least that is what I find myself thinking when I repeat certain patterns as if I'm one of Pavlov's dogs.

The exciting thing is, just as a computer can be reprogrammed, *your "tapes" can be "reprogrammed."* One way of thinking about it is you can place the old beliefs in the "trash bin," letting go of those that don't serve and are hurting you. You then add new "software" (beliefs), writing a program that makes for a more enjoyable life.

The truth is we all have beliefs that hold us back.

Initially, you learn PSCYH-K by attending a workshop. If you would like to go to a trained practitioner for private sessions, you have this option too.

I have utilized this tool myself. I only recommend things to my readers that I've personally experienced and feel have been of benefit. It is wonderful that we can *choose* to continue to grow our whole lives. *Will you intend this for yourself?*

You Can't Change What You Don't Know

The thing is, *you cannot re-program a limiting or hurtful belief if you don't know you have it.* This is where PSYCH-K comes in. PSYCH-K uses **muscle testing** to access your unconscious beliefs.

You can test your response to a belief easily and immediately. Your body knows! In this way, *you can access your unconscious beliefs and then use a simple process to change them to more self-affirming beliefs.*

PSYCH-K shows you how to access your unconscious beliefs and provides tools to re-program the new beliefs you'd like to hold. The process involves balancing both sides of the brain for whole brain integration. Whole brain integration benefits you immensely.

You can address a belief and perform a balancing in just a few moments. You then muscle test the new belief and when it tests "strong" you know you have been successful.

Complex issues may require several sessions to balance as there may be many aspects to them (for example self-esteem issues). In these cases it may be beneficial to consult with a practitioner, although you can also work with complex issues on your own.

PSCYH-K can be a great tool to process your feelings and beliefs about your body. As you practice changing your beliefs, you simply proceed with your life and *in a short time (changing several beliefs) you watch your life change—sometimes dramatically.*

The great thing is, as with EFT, you can learn PSYCH-K easily and use it yourself after a brief period of training in the technique. That means you don't have to go to an expert and shell out lots of money to improve your life.

PSYCH-K allows you to be an *active participant* in your own change process because it teaches you how to use the technique. How good is that! You can use it in the privacy of your own home.

I've offered a brief explanation of PSYCH-K. It's not meant to be exhaustive. Check it out and play with it.

Here's the website:

http://dev.psych-k.com and/or the book: http://amzn.to/PSYCH-K.

The website will let you know where workshops are being held near you (the initial workshop is two days and is really fun). The book doesn't really describe the process itself. The workshop introduces you to the techniques and gives you hands-on experience with them. You may then utilize these techniques on your own.

I hope you enjoy. And remember, although it's a remarkable tool, *you need to use it in order for it to work!*

Important Note:

EFT and PSYCH-K are not replacements for professional help. If you have a condition that warrants medical or psychiatric care, seek the advice of your medical doctor or mental health practitioner.

I am not an affiliate and do not receive compensation in any way for either EFT or PSYCH-K. *The point is to turn you on to amazing, fun, tools to improve your life.*

CONCLUSIONS

Look at every path closely and deliberately.
Try it as many times as you think necessary. Then ask yourself alone,
one question . . . Does this path have heart? For me there is only the traveling
on paths that have heart, on any path that may have heart,
and the only worthwhile challenge is to traverse its full length—
and there I travel, looking, looking breathlessly.

—Don Juan

You Are God To Your Cells

A friend said something to me recently that I found both beautiful and fascinating. He said that *we are god to the cells of our body.* In other words, our cells completely rely upon us to love and take good care of them. They look to us. They need us. Recall Dr. Lipton's research and his conclusion that love is the most powerful thing we can do for our cells. *Our body needs us to love it.*

It is my sincere hope that you have benefitted tremendously from *FIL*. I envision that you're feeling better about your body and your life. I imagine good things entering your life as a result and I hope you do too.

Although you may slip back into old patterns on occasion, as I do, you now know how to get back into a good feeling state relative to your body. The same principles can be applied to other areas of your life as well. It becomes easier and easier the more you reinforce it.

> **Thank your body daily for all the functions it performs in order to keep you moving through and enjoying your life. Remain aware of the fact that your body gives you life and every experience you get to have is because you have a body.**

If you have daughters, I believe one of the best gifts you can give them is your increased love of your own body. What a great example for them. As they see you loving your body more, they will likely incorporate some of these positive feelings toward their own bodies.

Perhaps within the span of a generation, there will be a significant shift in how women perceive and respond to their bodies. My hope is that women will befriend their bodies, as I hope you have as a result of *The Fall In Love Body Program.*

In doing so, a deep healing will take place. While we cannot save the world, we can engage in falling more in love with our own bodies and ourselves. Change happens one person at a time. Now is the time to begin.

Really, *The Fall In Love Body Program* is about self-love. It's about learning how not to sell ourselves out, how not to betray ourselves as women.

Contrary to being selfish, caring for yourself is the most reverential action you can take. Caring for and loving yourself provides a foundation for caring and loving others and being loved. It promotes a healthy sense of self-esteem.

I trust that if you have utilized *The Fall In Love Body Program* you are loving yourself more.

Remember, love and happiness are a state of mind and are not reserved for a particular body type. The best thing you can do for yourself is live a life that is true to who you are and follow a path with heart.

The Answers Lie Within:
The Gods on Mount Olympus Hide The Secret of Life

There is a story about the Greek gods on Mount Olympus. Having created the earth and all that was upon it, they had one further task to accomplish. They had to hide the secret of life where it could not be found until humans had evolved in consciousness and were ready to receive the information.

The gods argued about where to hide the secret of life. One suggested the highest mountain, another the deepest ocean. Finally, one of the gods came up with the solution. He suggested hiding it in the last place humans would look, the place they would explore only after all other possibilities had been exhausted—in the human heart.

The answers lie within our hearts, within our true nature. The most profound truths are often the simplest. The knowledge that we seek is inside.

Still, it is good to have a flashlight at times to light the way. I hope this program has provided the opportunity to shine a light toward a path that leads to you and your body becoming the best of friends.

Peace and blessings to you on that path and be well until we meet again.

RESOURCES

B elow are a few resources that have been favorites of mine. Aside from the general bodywork portion, all the other resources have been utilized by me and have provided remarkable information or results.

I am not an affiliate and do not receive any benefit from referring you to these tools and sites. The intention is to provide you with great tools for your personal growth and well-being. They are not intended to replace medical treatment or traditional therapy.

Bodywork

The free dictionary defines bodywork as a general term for therapeutic methods that center on the body for the promotion of physical health and emotional and spiritual well-being, including massage, various systems of touch and manipulation, relaxation techniques, and practices designed to affect the body's energy flow.

Today we have many types and forms of bodywork available to choose from. Massage is a great way to relax and is especially beneficial if you are living a stressful lifestyle. In any event, it is a wonderful modality and feels great. Deep tissue massage is beneficial on many levels.

Meditation and Yoga are wonderful tools for overall well-being. It's easy to find locations near you by checking on-line. You can also do a Google search on Bodywork for further information.

Mystery Of Healing Tapes—by Candida Condor

I have had remarkable experiences with these tapes. Dr. Condor has expanded these tapes and the program is now called: ***Engaging The Healer Within***. They are by far my favorite healing tapes. I could tell some stories! I cannot overemphasize how valuable these tapes have been. The series includes relaxation sessions. Amazing!

www.drcondor.com

Click on the *Engaging The Healer Within* Series. At this time it appears Dr. Condor is in process of updating her website and a link to purchase this series doesn't appear to be available at the moment. The series is excellent and I'm still including it so you may have access when it's completed.

Devotional Music & Chanting

My favorite devotional music is produced by Snatam Kaur. Her voice is angelic. Listening to devotional music and chanting is a wonderful way to experience a sense of calm and well-being. You can play it in the background when you're at home or listen while in your car. There is a large selection of various artists and their on-line sites have samples of music you can listen to.

http://www.snatamkaur.com

David Wolfe—Health, Nutrition, & Longevity

David Wolfe's Longevity Conferences are awesome. He provides cutting edge speakers and information in the field of nutrition, wellness, and longevity. If you sign up to receive information, he sends lots of videos on a great variety of health-related topics. Numerous YouTube videos are posted as well.

http://www.thelongevitynowconference.com

the Fall in Love Process
www.thefallinloveprocess.com
120

The Biology Of Belief—Dr. Bruce Lipton

In addition to interviews on-line, Dr. Lipton has several fascinating books, including *The Biology of Belief: Unleashing the Power of Consciousness, Matter & Miracles.*

http://www.brucelipton.com

Why People Don't Heal—Caroline Myss

Caroline Myss' *Why People Don't Heal* is a profound tool for understanding the victim/martyr role. This tool is about self-empowerment. *Why People Don't Heal* is available in book form and audio tapes. You can order them through Amazon or her website. Myss' website offers a wealth of information and additional products.

http://www.myss.com

Abraham-Hicks

The Abraham-Hicks website offers incredible tools to access your own inner guidance through observing your emotions and working with them. Esther Hicks created the concept that the reason we want anything is that we believe we will feel better in the having of that thing. Abe-Hicks is a beacon for self-empowerment and creating a joyous and fun-filled life. They have numerous books, CDs and audios.

My personal favorite book is *Ask and It Is Given*. **Ask and It Is Given provides 22 remarkable processes you can use to improve your life.** Check out the *Rampage of Appreciation* process. It changed my life.

Additionally, you can order their monthly CDs, attend a workshop near you, or receive their daily quotes. Phenomenal information. Their website contains videos and lots of information.

http://www.abraham-hicks.com

Esalen—the best place on the planet!

Esalen is nestled along the coast of Big Sur and has been providing workshops and retreats since the 1960's. Their beautiful natural spring hot tubs are on the cliffs overlooking the ocean and are open 24-hours daily. Meals are prepared from their huge organic garden. In addition to participating in a wide variety of workshops, personal retreats are available (my favorite way to go). You can't imagine unless you've been there.

Esalen provides many mind-body and healing modalities in their workshops and massages (overlooking the ocean!) are available.

As noted on their website:

The Esalen Institute was founded in 1962 as an alternative educational center devoted to the exploration of what Aldous Huxley called the "human potential"—the world of unrealized human capacities that lies beyond the imagination. Esalen soon became known for its blend of East/ West philosophies, its experiential/ didactic workshops, the steady influx of philosophers, psychologists, artists, and religious thinkers, and its breathtaking grounds and natural hot springs.

Check out this remarkable place:

http://www.esalen.org

APPENDIX A

The Exercises

How To Do The Core Exercises:

At the beginning of each exercise I will explain how to do it and will provide at least one example. You may customize it to what works for you. There is no right or wrong, but it is important to hold to the basic concept of the exercise.

Do not judge yourself as you are writing. Just let it flow. You may repeat many of the same things over and over and that is fine. Add new things as well.

Most importantly, you need to actually do the exercises for them to work.

Core Exercise One:
Everything I Experienced Today

Note: If you can do only one exercise do this one. *This exercise is what in itself created a massive shift in me relative to how I felt about my body.* Do not underestimate this exercise.

If you did not read the book or do any other exercises, this first exercise in itself can promote tremendous change in relation to your feelings about your body. Do it!

The Practice:

For at least 30 days perform this as a written exercise daily. You may choose the time of day. It is best if you can be fairly consistent regarding the time of day, only because if you are in a routine in this regard it can help to ensure that you continue with the process.

If you cannot perform the exercise at approximately the same time daily, that is all right. Do it any time during the day or evening that works for you; however, do it each day for the 30-day period.

After 30 days you may continue to write this exercise daily or you may perform it mentally as you are going about your day. You can easily do the exercise mentally while you are involved in your daily routine. In fact, it is great if you can do it mentally several times a day. Initially, though, it is best to write it as well. It helps you incorporate these new thoughts and feelings about your body and plants new seeds within you about your body.

The intention is that at some point these new thoughts and feelings will become second nature to you. The new beliefs reflected in the

124
the Fall in Love Process
www.thefallinloveprocess.com

practice become dominant and take the place of older negative thoughts, feelings, and beliefs that do not serve you. At the least, they begin to form the majority of your thoughts and feelings about your body, so when past negative thoughts, feelings, or beliefs arise they can quickly be replaced with the more positive reflections and emotions that have been cultivated by practicing this exercise.

The Exercise:

Take a few moments to reflect upon your day today. It is best to do this particular exercise in the evening since you are reflecting back upon the day; however, if morning is the only convenient time for you to perform this exercise, reflect upon the prior day.

Set a daily intention, however, first thing in the morning, that as you go through your day you will notice things in a different way. Also, **as you are experiencing your day or reflecting back upon it, keep this thought in mind: that everything you are experiencing or did experience in your day is because you have a body.**

Become aware of the people you encounter, pleasant exchanges, or a pleasing moment. Notice things that you enjoyed or are in the process of enjoying. It can be interactions with friends, family, strangers, co-workers, and kindnesses you observe or experience. You might realize how much you enjoyed the taste of a meal or the companionship of a friend or family member.

It may be that a particular sight such as the ocean or a sunset might have brought a sense of joy. Perhaps you enjoyed a beautiful scene in nature or an activity. Maybe you saw a beautiful mountain, a body of water, a piece of music, a book, shopping, seeing a film or play, tasting great food or wine, a child's smile, laughing with a friend, making love, dancing, laughing hilariously, riding your bike. **Notice anything that feels good to you. It does not matter what it is. What is important is the feeling it evokes.**

Spend a few moments writing down some of these experiences. **Write until you feel a sense of well-being. Connect this feeling of well-being to an appreciation of your body that allowed you to have these experiences.**

Realize that without your body you would not have experienced **any** of these things that have brought you a sense of joy or satisfaction. If this does not occur in the beginning stages of your writing, hang in there. Over time your sense of well-being is likely to increase significantly.

An additional benefit of performing this exercise is that you will begin to gain a greater appreciation of how many things you experience in a day that feel good to you.

Appreciation is one of the most powerful, life-changing experiences you can cultivate. This exercise will help you to do that.

After writing, look over what you have written and **allow the good feelings to re-enter your awareness**. Again, realize that none of this would have been possible without your body. Being in your body has enabled you to have these experiences.

Do not skip over this exercise or dismiss it as too simple or basic to be effective. It is the single most effective and important part of the FIL Body Program.

The most profound things are sometimes right before our eyes but we overlook them due to their simplicity. Part of the beauty of The Fall In Love Program lies in its simplicity, yet it is profound in its ability to create an awakening in you. (See the story at the end about the gods on Mount Olympus.)

Your heart has waited a long time for this awakening. Claim it for yourself now!

Example:

I had such a great time with my friend today. Our conversation felt so fun and nurturing. One of the best moments was when the most lovely little girl came over to me at the coffeehouse and stared at me with her huge brown eyes. She would leave and a few moments later return and stay longer. The next thing I knew she was planted in my lap. We played on my computer looking at animals. Just being at the coffeehouse and seeing familiar faces and talking with acquaintances and friends was really fun. The sunset was gorgeous tonight. I love how the sun reflected in the water. I could look at it forever and melt into the feeling of peace and tranquility that I experience at this time of day. Watching day turn to night, today, was great. I absolutely come alive at dusk and I love the feeling of it. I loved that I could hear the ocean from my home today and I started my day by lying in bed and listening to it. What a great way to awaken. I enjoyed delicious organic food today. I love to eat things that taste wonderful and feel good in my body. I was able to talk with my mom today and I love the sound of her voice "lighting up" when she hears it is me on the other end of the line. This evening I spent some time reading the most delightful book. The feeling of the warm shower tonight was delicious. As I reflect on all these things I enjoyed today, I realize that none of it would have been possible without my body.

Everything I experienced today is because I have a body. Good experiences I had today.

_____

_____

_____

_____

_____

_____

_____

_____

Core Exercise Two:
My Body And All It Does For Me

The Practice:

Perform this as a written exercise daily for at least 30 days. As with the first exercise, after 30 days you may either continue to write it or do it only mentally. Within the first 30 days try to practice it mentally throughout the day as well, as you notice all the things your body does for you. Feel your appreciation.

You may do this as a written exercise any time of day or night. It is best to do these written exercises around the same time of day if you can.

The Exercise:

All My Body Does For Me: Write about your body in such a way that you acknowledge all it does for you.

Make it positive. Do not think too hard about this—just let it flow. If initially you cannot think of anything, stay with it until you can think of at least one thing. As you progress through your days, you will be able to add to your list.

Read the material in this book for inspiration if you become stuck, and access the Fall In Love Process website for support at www. fallinloveprocess.com.

After you write this exercise each day, go back and read it out loud to yourself. Write and read it until you *experience a good feeling* about your body.

The following are two examples that I wrote. These are offered to give you an idea how to go about this exercise. Yours will be unique to you, as mine is to me. It does not have to be in complete sentences or grammatically correct. There is no right or wrong.

Example One:

My lovely, magnificent body, that contains my heart and soul and spirit. My unique body. All of who I am is experienced through this magnificent body which functions with the utmost precision, more intricate than the most sophisticated computer. I adore my body, with all it is and does. All the factors that come together in order for me to talk, walk, think, feel, intuit, process, observe, emote, fly, move, toward the greatest heights of ecstasy, joy, tears, belly laughs, sighs, whispers, love-making, romping, skipping, dancing, driving, moving, stillness, giggles, singing, jumping, yelping . . . on and on . . . all of it, me, us, existing, thriving, meticulously working for me, more finely tuned than a Swiss watch, working seemingly effortlessly for me to be here in ME, here on this fabulous, beautiful earth . . . LIVING!

Example Two:

My body. How wonderful and marvelous IT is! There is nothing like it in all the Universe. My body can so easily come into perfect alignment. It wants to! My body is already doing so well and all is aligning for it, me, to feel even better and better. My body is really happy. I can feel its tremendous happiness. My body thrives and plays. My body loves to touch and be touched. My body functions impeccably in hundreds of thousands of ways. Wow! My body takes me everywhere I go and allows me every life experience. My body participates in every single experience I have. I would not be here if not for this magnificent body. Bodies are awesome. My body sings and dances. My body soars. My body rocks! My body brings me tremendous pleasure—and joy. My body is happy. My body has enabled me to walk, talk, taste, see, and hear today. Because of this I get to appreciate all the beautiful sights and wonders this life makes available. I am truly loving coming to love my body for the incredible opportunity it has afforded me to live this life so freely and unencumbered. It works so well. All is well in my body. My body is free. Life sure is good in this body!

My Body—and All It Does for Me

_____

_____

_____

_____

_____

_____

_____

_____

_____

_____

_____

_____

_____

_____

the Fall in Love Process
www.thefallinloveprocess.com
132

Core Exercise Three:
My Favorite Moments In Life

The Practice:

This is an exercise you will perform one time only. It is meant to be a written exercise. You may go back and add to it if you think of additional things you experienced in your life that you particularly enjoyed. Feel the good feelings that course through you as you reflect upon these moments. You may return to this document and read it out loud to yourself anytime. Feel free to add to it.

The Exercise:

Take a few moments to reflect upon some of your favorite moments in life. It may relate to an event, a place, a person, a conversation, an experience, or an activity. Now write down some of your best moments, the most memorable, those that have touched or impacted you deeply.

Write anything you think of that has cultivated a sense of joy or happiness. It may be a peak experience you had while in nature, a special love relationship or friendship, a conversation, your work, the birth of a child, a special recognition you received, offering service to others, making a special purchase. It doesn't matter what it is; rather, *it is the feeling it evoked in you that is significant.*

After you write about these special times and experiences, take a moment to read it aloud and reflect back upon what you have written. Read it over often as you use *The Fall In Love Body Program.* The purpose is to *re-create the emotion of the events or experiences,* to get in touch with feeling good.

As you are performing this exercise, and each time you read it over, **realize and affirm to yourself that without your body none of these experiences would have been possible. Reflect upon the fact that it was because of your body that you were able to have these moments.**

Example:

I love the times spent with my grandmother at the kitchen table. All the laughs we shared and the sweet conversation. Being with my family in Pennsylvania, our conversations and all the things we do together. Playing Scrabble with and going to lunch with my mom. Just being with her. Hanging out with my sister and our ritual of going shopping, which I love only because I am with her and she gets it that it is an act of love and enjoys "torturing" me by insisting on just one more store! Playing with my sweet German Shepherd Bacchus and watching his face smile and his tongue hang out. All the wonderful moments with friends and loves, the feeling of warmth, support, fun, playfulness, genuineness, love, irreverence, and joy. Knowing I have such great people in my life and such love. Moments with my father on his porch at night in Costa Rica listening to his great life stories. Early mornings when he would toss pebbles on the tin roof of my cabin to awaken me and then tease me as I walked up the path to his house saying he thought I was never going to get up—at about 6:30 am. The beautiful birds that would come in the morning to feed and the sound of the monkeys calling out from the mountain. Holding newborn and little babies. Being with my nephews and niece and my friends' children, and how great it is being loved and loving children as they grow through each stage of life. Accompanying my nephew on late night walks year after year when I visit and camping out together in the same room. Having big squirt gun battles with my little nephew and getting soaked. Jumping on the trampoline with him, tickling, and playing basketball and football. Giving my commencement speech on the topic of A Different Drummer about individuality and developing your own path. Looking back and realizing I have lived my life in this way. Providing workshops and interacting with others in a

134
the Fall in Love Process
www.thefallinloveprocess.com

way that feeds my soul and spirit. Sharing my personal experiences, easy and painful, and using them as a stepping stone to a more wonderful perspective. All the times in and at the ocean which creates such joy in me that it takes my breath away. My travels through the United States, Europe, Tahiti, Hawaii, the Caribbean. Driving up the northern California coast. Esalen at Big Sur, especially the hot tubs on the cliffs overlooking the ocean and their amazing organic food freshly grown in their gardens and the incredible beauty that stuns me every single time. Gazing into the night sky with all the stars and wondering about the mystery and magic of life. Experiencing a connection with it all. Feeling the oneness, the love. Marveling that love is the most powerful force and presence in the universe.

My Favorite Moments In Life

Anchoring

A way that you can increase the effectiveness of these exercises is to use a simple technique called **anchoring.** Anchoring is a way to form an association in your neurology, your body, that expands upon your good feelings.

As you are performing an exercise and at a time when you are feeling good, charged, positive, do something with your body that will anchor the feeling.

Anchoring is a tool that I believe was first developed in the field of neuro-linguistic programming. Anthony Robbins has also utilized this technique in simple, yet effective, ways.

Here's an example of anchoring. When you are in this state of feeling really good (about your body), reach down and touch the points of your thumb and middle finger together. Do this a few times when you are in this good feeling state. You will then notice that all you have to do is put those two fingers together in this way and you will feel the good feeling!

The fact that this works demonstrates the amazing wonder of our bodies and is just one of many examples of the mind-body connection. I like to touch my inner arm to anchor in a state. You can anchor more than one state by using various parts of the body.

If it starts to lose its effectiveness, begin again and repeat the process when you are in a state of feeling great. You want to feel as good as you can when you "anchor" in your feelings, as the better you feel the more effective and powerful it will be.

FIL RESOURCES

The Fall In Love Process Website

Perhaps after reading and using *The Fall In Love Body Program* you feel you have taken great strides towards loving your body and you are satisfied. Some people may find they would like to take it a step further, continue their FIL Process, and be connected with a community of like-minded individuals.

The Fall In Love Process includes more than this book. The Fall In Love Process website is a place where you can visit as often as you would like for support and to reinforce your new perspective on your body and your life.

In addition to the body program, *The Fall In Love Process* includes learning to love yourself, create loving relationships, and if applicable, making your way through a break-up in a way that empowers and strengthens you.

Book Two in *The Fall In Love Series* is the **Relationship Program.** Several years ago I had a date that culminated in another one of those "aha" moments. I realized that by mid-life people still long for love, yet often they no longer believe it's possible. Think: painful past relationship experiences. This creates quite a dilemma. **The Relationship Program** guides you out of that painful dilemma and into a more healthy way of viewing and experiencing relationships.

Book Three is The Break-Up Program. It leads you through the difficult process of a separation, utilizing it as a window of opportunity for personal transformation.

In order to assist you, and because it brings me joy, you can interact with myself and others who are engaged in *The Fall In Love Process*.

The Fall In Love Process website will include courses, posts, videos, and audios.

The nature of the website may change at my discretion and as I learn what you want most.

To Fall In Love: www.thefallinloveprocess.com

I think of FIL as a movement. Its time has come. I invite you to participate in this process with others who are choosing to empower their lives by supporting one another in learning to love your bodies and your selves.

ABOUT THE AUTHOR

D r. Thomas has been involved in the personal growth and transformation arena for over 30 years. Her engaging presentation style has made her a favorite of audiences. She presents workshops and leads therapeutic intensive processes throughout the United States.

The author holds a doctorate in clinical psychology, and two master's degrees. She believes that personal life experience is the greatest teacher and all her programs and workshops are a result of her own life experiences. Her desire is to help others reach their fullest potential and live a joyful and authentic life.

Websites are: thefallinloveprocess.com and bestrelationshipsever.com.

Dr. Thomas currently resides near San Diego, California.

Contact The Author

To contact the author regarding speaking engagements, workshops, or personal mentoring: email: lauren@thefallinloveprocess.com or call: 760-487-8016

You may also choose to interact on the main website at:

the Fall in Love Process
www.thefallinloveprocess.com